Toilet Adoption in Rural India

This book examines sanitation and toilet access across rural India, focusing on psychological, sociocultural, infrastructural, and normative barriers to the initiative of the Swachh Bharat Mission (SBM). While sketching the evolution of sanitation policies in India, it assesses their impact on sanitation behaviour. It also studies the implications of variations in caste, religion, and geography on toilet usage across Indian states.

By analysing data from various states and intensive micro-level studies of three states, i.e., rural Bihar, Gujarat, and Telangana, this volume:

- Suggests that sociocultural factors are as significant as economic factors in shaping sanitation behaviour;
- Argues that the concepts of cleanliness and pollution are often determined by the social-cultural context, rooted in historical events that have shaped traditional beliefs and ideas about space;
- Explores gendered perspectives on the usage of and access to toilets;
- Highlights the limited effectiveness of Information, Education, and Communication (IEC) programmes in encouraging toilet adoption and emphasises the need for information dissemination at the ground level; and
- Gives recommendations for enhancing the adoption of toilets in rural India, including provision for more than one toilet per household, uninterrupted access to water, and behavioural change to combat open defecation.

This book will be useful for students studying sociology, psychology, social work, and development studies. It will also be an invaluable companion to NGOs, social workers, and activists actively involved in water, sanitation, and hygiene. Moreover, this book holds immense value as a pivotal resource and point of reference for policymakers engaged in rural development with a specific focus on Sustainable Development Goals.

Saswata Narayan Biswas is Professor at the Institute of Rural Management Anand (IRMA), India.

Indranil De is Professor at the Institute of Rural Management Anand (IRMA), India.

Gyan Mudra is Professor and Chairperson at the School of Gender Studies, Tata Institute of Social Sciences (TISS), Hyderabad, India.

Deepa Gupta is a Doctoral fellow at the Institute of Rural Management Anand (IRMA), India.

Toilet Adoption in Rural India

Social Norms and Behavioural Changes

Saswata Narayan Biswas, Indranil De, Gyan Mudra, and Deepa Gupta

Routledge
Taylor & Francis Group
LONDON AND NEW YORK

First published 2024
by Routledge
4 Park Square, Milton Park, Abingdon, Oxon OX14 4RN

and by Routledge
605 Third Avenue, New York, NY 10158

Routledge is an imprint of the Taylor & Francis Group, an informa business

British Library Cataloguing-in-Publication Data
A catalogue record for this book is available from the British Library

ISBN: 978-1-032-55496-9 (hbk)
ISBN: 978-1-032-72625-0 (pbk)
ISBN: 978-1-032-72626-7 (ebk)

DOI: 10.4324/9781032726267

Typeset in Times New Roman
by Deanta Global Publishing Services, Chennai, India

Contents

Figures

Tables

Acknowledgements

Sanitation and hygiene are the bedrock of a physically healthy community and society. Removing human waste and keeping it at harm's bay has been a concern of all societies since the dawn of civilisation (i.e. Harappa and Mohenjo-Daro). Similarly, cleaning the body and performing daily ablutions have been part of Indian society since the Vedic period, when personal hygiene or daily baths were absent in many parts of the world. But, because of a complex interaction of poverty, population, and notions of pollution, the basic concepts of sanitation and hygiene got obliterated by the convoluted notions of purity and pollution that emerged with time. The lack of physical infrastructure for sanitation was perpetuated and justified through a misrepresented cultural interpretation that Indians preferred open defecation. Under this pretext, millions of people were allowed to languish in unsanitary and unhealthy conditions affecting both the physical and psychological well-being of individuals, affecting the nation's growth. Despite the critical nature of sanitation, very few scholarly studies have emerged on sanitation in India. This book attempts to fill this gap by exploring toilet adoption's economic, social, and psychological aspects in rural India.

A book of this nature would not have been possible without the support of many people and institutions. At the outset, we express our gratitude to the National Institute of Rural Development and Panchayati Raj (NIRD&PR) for supporting part of the study through their research grant to the Institute of Rural Management Anand (IRMA). We thank the Institute of Rural Management Anand (IRMA) for facilitating and supporting this work. We are thankful to the IRMA library for their unstinted effort in providing bibliographic support services, allowing us to go through the archives, and helping us to go through the student projects over the last 25 years. Without the help of the respective district administration, it would not have been possible to access ground-level primary and district-level data; we thank all of them for their kind help. We are thankful to all the participants of our studies across the country for being incredibly supportive and candid with us. Without them, this work would not have been possible.

1 Sanitation and Well-Being

Sanitation is essential to physical and psychological well-being. It is critical in developing human capability and human capital. In 2015, the United Nations acknowledged sanitation as a human right. It included sanitation as one of the sustainable development goals (SDGs) to achieve all of humanity's physical, mental, and social well-being. India is one of the countries committed to achieving the 17 SDGs of the United Nations by 2030. The challenge for India was gigantic. While there was a consistent push to improve sanitation in urban India, rural India having about 68% of the total population had remained in relative neglect. In 2001 about 22% of rural households had a toilet at home (Kumar, 2015). After about a decade of the Total Sanitation Campaign (TSC) in 2011, slightly over 30% of rural households owned a toilet. Thus, a large proportion of the rural population continued open defecation. There is strong evidence that open defecation has both health- and non-health-related adverse outcomes, which have long-term consequences for a nation and the world. The impact of sanitation coverage on health primarily relates to anaemia, diarrhoea leading to poor nutrition, and stunting. Open defecation has substantial negative psychological consequences for women besides health and hygiene issues. The lack of toilets for girls in schools is one of the critical reasons for girl students dropping out of school and the gender gap. The multifaceted negative impact of open defecation has been thoroughly explored in recent years, and the results are scary.

A systematic review exploring the relationship between sanitation and mental and social well-being examined the full text of 738 studies published in various journals (Sclar et al., 2018). The analysis revealed that sanitation impacts individuals' and communities' health status and has an adverse psychological impact. Open defecation has grave consequences on women's physical and mental health. Their analysis of published papers showed that women have been at the receiving end of open defecation. Many women reported that they experienced non-partner sexual violence, stress, and anxiety due to open defecation. The women experienced the loss of dignity, privacy, shame, embarrassment, and fear of being assaulted during open defecation. Such experiences of self or shared experience of group members induced anxiety and fear every time one had to defecate in the open and thus leading to mental health problems and the attendant health hazards. Therefore, open defecation is related to physical and mental health and increases gender inequality. They also pointed out that public sanitation facilities have similar attributes of

DOI: 10.4324/9781032726267-1

being unsafe, insecure, and lacking in privacy because of their non-gender-sensitive design and location. Most public sanitation facilities for women lack doors or have broken doors with no locks, low walls, and poor lighting, compromising the safety and privacy of women (Sclar et al., 2018). These studies have demonstrated that lack of sanitation spreads infectious diseases like diarrhoea and affects the mental health of individuals and communities. Scalar and his associates developed a model based on their systematic review, illustrating the perceived threats from open defecation and public toilets, particularly to women. The two significant risks identified were a perceived lack of privacy and safety. Many women perceive that defecating in the open is likely to get them assaulted verbally, physically, and sexually. The study observed that toilets at home do not permanently alleviate the perceived fear of using the toilet. It was the design and location of the toilets that mattered. The significant barriers to safety perception were toilets with low walls, no roof, door locks, poor lighting, slippery floors, etc.

Open Defecation and Health

The 'Asian enigma' is a term coined by Spears (Spears, 2020) to underline the paradox confronting developmental economists and social scientists worldwide. The paradox centres around the fact that despite having almost double the per capita GDP (in PPP terms) compared to sub-Saharan Africa (World Bank, u.d.), Indian children are shorter. In other words, Indian children have stunted growth. Stunting refers to children's impaired growth. Technically stunting is when children's height for age is greater than two standard deviations below the World Health Organization's (WHO) Child Growth Standards median. Spears argues that stunting in India results from a higher density of open defecation than in sub-Saharan Africa. Recent research has suggested that early childhood physical growth is related to physical strength in later stages of life; it is also linked to children's cognitive abilities. Studies have pointed out that early childhood stunting adversely affects the child's cognitive development, impairing their ability to perform effectively in later life. A study conducted in India, Bangladesh, Brazil, Nepal, Peru, and Pakistan suggested that early-life bacterial and viral pathogen burden is associated with cognitive development at age five. It was also found that iron deficiency anaemia during early childhood leads to poor cognitive abilities later in life (Alam et al., 2020).

Diarrhoea kills over half a million children annually. It is the second leading cause of death for children under five (World Health Organization, 2009). The National Family Health Survey (NFHS) indicates that diarrhoea among children increased from 9% in 2016 to 9.2% in 2020. The United Nations International Children's Emergency Fund (UNICEF) reports that most deaths of children under five are caused by malnourishment (45%), followed by pneumonia (15%) and diarrhoea (8%). It should also be noted that malnourishment is partly caused by diarrhoea due to poor hygiene and sanitation. The nutritional status of minor children worsens with water contaminated with human faeces from sewage septic tanks and open defecation.

Despite rapid economic growth during the first decade of this millennium, the primary sanitation conditions had remained dismal. More than half the population did not have access to basic toilet facilities, resulting in diseases affecting children. One of the goals of sustainable development by the United Nations was to provide basic sanitation and access to water to all people by 2030. Sanitation and water are the two vital elements that contribute to the creation of human capital. One of the most extensive intervention programmes in sanitation was launched by the prime minister of India, Shri Narendra Modi, in October 2014, with the boldest declaration that India would be free of open defecation by October 2019. The first step was creating a facilitative condition by constructing toilets. The intervention increased coverage exponentially and brought toilets to the homes of around 96.5% of the people.

Sanitation and Human Capability

The human capability approach pioneered by Amartya Sen and advanced by Martha Nussbaum has been around for over three decades. It rests on two fundamental resources: health and education. Good health at a younger age is also a prerequisite for developing effective learning capabilities. Health does not mean the absence of disease. A healthy person enjoys complete physical, mental, and social well-being (Callahan, 1973). Human capability increases when individuals experience complete health and are not just free from disease and infirmity. Appreciation of the fact that health contributes to people's overall well-being has been highlighted in several studies. Studies have documented how sanitation influences health that transcends disease and affects the overall development of society. Sanitation is linked to children's educational attainment in many countries, instrumental in widening the gender gap. For example, studies in Africa and Asia have pointed out that the lack of toilets in schools has caused girl children to drop out of the school system (Caruso et al., 2018).

Studies have considered the role of human capability and its transformation into human capital at the core of any development phenomenon. Nations often falter in their developmental trajectory because the essential factors are often overlooked while focussing on other factors. There is enough evidence in the literature to suggest the importance of early childhood in determining adult capabilities of cognition, motivation, and health (Heckman, 2007). Given that earnings are also a function of physical and mental abilities, thus childhood stunting affects the potential for future earnings adversely (Scholder et al., 2013). Human capital is the most critical element in productivity in any nation, depending on an individual's physical and cognitive abilities. A nation that wants to progress must take care of the early childhood development of its citizens. Open defecation is the single reason for early childhood stunting in India (Spears et al., 2013). The impact of stunting on the economy has interested many researchers. In one study, Spears and his colleagues used existing data sets from 112 districts in India; statistical analysis of the data suggested that districts with a higher density of open defecation had a higher degree of stunting (Spears et al., 2013). John Hoddinott from the International

Food Policy Research Institute, Washington (DC), and his colleagues reviewed the research on stunting. Their analysis suggests that lack of growth in early childhood results in loss of height in adulthood. They quote research suggesting that a 1% rise in height leads to a 2.4% rise in income. They suggested that attained height is a proxy measure for several dimensions of human capital social skills, cognitive abilities, social class, and overall health parameters. The data from Congo, India, and Bangladesh estimated the average benefit-cost of interventions for stunting at 3.8, 34.1, and 18, respectively, for the three countries. In the case of India, the benefit stands out astoundingly high at 34.1 compared to the other two countries (Hoddinott et al., 2013).

Gender Inequality and Sanitation

Inadequate provision for maintenance of toilets and the toilet's physical location often deter women from using them. Therefore, policymakers must examine the structural, environmental, and social factors inhibiting toilet use. For example, one may consider that toilets at home may provide women with privacy and safety; however, structural and cultural issues may prevent women from enjoying privacy and safety. Thus, there is a need to explore ways to mitigate these factors from the users' perspective, specifically essential for a woman. These studies infer that the toilet's construction can also lead to gender discrimination and potentially increase the gender gap. In other related studies, it has been found that poor sanitation is associated with high maternal mortality and adverse pregnancy outcomes, resulting in more significant psychosocial stress among women (Caruso et al., 2018).

Interestingly, while a functional household toilet was related to better psychological well-being, access to self had no relationship with anxiety and depression. The women experienced insecurity, anxiety, and stress while defecating in a functional toilet when the toilets were not appropriately designed. Therefore, open defecation and poorly designed toilets had differential impacts on men and women. Access to a toilet facility may not reduce the perceived threats to women. Enough conditions should be there to make them feel safe. Because of many sociocultural reasons, one cannot assume that toilet access will result in their usage. The only condition for better mental health status for women is the experience of safety and security has to be there; it is pointed out that mental health is a significant factor in reducing desirability. The mental health burden has been increasing over the years. It has economic consequences; therefore, the construction of toilets cannot be the end-all or all of sanitation. We must create conditions where both men and women can access and use toilets without the negative psychological consequences discussed here.

Apart from stunting, open defecation substantially impacts diarrhoeal diseases related to poor hand hygiene and lack of water. Researchers observe some chronic health effects of open defecation, such as anaemia, giardiasis, and stunting accompanying impaired cognition. For children under five, diarrhoea ranks second on the list of causes of death (WHO, 2017). More than half a million children die due to diarrhoea worldwide. It is also a significant cause of malnutrition. The major causes of diarrhoea among children in rural India have been open defecation, lack of water, and lack of hand hygiene. It is estimated that about 600 million people defecate in the open in India. Sanitation coverage in India is substantially lower than in other developing nations. The National Sample Survey (NSS) 2012 revealed that 59.4% of households in rural India do not have any toilet facilities. Lack of sanitation contributes to about 10% of the disease burden worldwide, including diarrhoea and stunting (Mara et al., 2010; Schmidt, 2014). India shares 38% of the global burden of stunted children, according to an estimate by UNICEF in 2011. The alarming situation in India is that about half (48%) of children under five years of age have stunted growth.

The positive impact of an open defecation-free (ODF) village is realised when everyone uses the toilet. Gertler and his colleagues estimated that the total elimination of open defecation in an area where everyone defecates openly increases the child's height by 0.44 standard deviations (Gertler et al., 2015). Therefore, partial elimination of open defecation does not significantly affect health status. However, at multiple levels, sanitation behaviour results from a complex decision-making process (e.g. individuals, households, community). The decision to have a toilet within the home is a household-level decision. Still, this decision is not just constrained by the availability of money but also by religious beliefs, the notion of purity, and how the neighbour will perceive it. The individual's decision to use the toilet may get determined by the gender and position of the person within the household. Coffey and his colleagues found that the revealed preference was for open defecation in rural north India and at least one member of 40% of the households with a functional working toilet defecated in the open (Coffey et al., 2014).

Therefore, a decisive intervention for improving access to sanitation is imperative.

> The right to sanitation was implicit in most other rights that preceded it, but much remains to be done so that every human being is able to defecate safely and without discrimination, wash oneself and one's hands after defecation, bathe and manage one's menstruation with safety, dignity, and privacy.
>
> (Patkar, 2016, p. 268)

Sanitation Behaviour and Culture

Past research on sanitation had primarily focused on lack of accessibility, like not having a toilet at home because of financial constraints at the household level, lack of proper public infrastructure, and social influence. Only a handful of studies have focused on sociocultural dimensions, such as social norms and religious values (Vyas & Spears, 2018). Religion often influences individuals' notions of purity and the concept of pollution. For example, the traditional caste system in India had created the notions of purity arranged hierarchically along the caste hierarchy. The Brahmins were considered the purest of all castes and Shudras at the bottom rung of purity, relegating them to perform all the tasks considered polluting, including removing the animal carcass and human excreta. Thus, sanitation in India has been traditionally related to religious practices. Among many social reformers, Gandhi recognised the relationship between sanitation and caste. He coined a respectful term for the lowest rung of the society and urged everybody to clean their excreta irrespective of their caste; as usual, Gandhi's call had met stiff resistance from the upper caste. The tradition of caste hierarchy and notions of purity and pollution have changed in the urban areas, perhaps because migrants predominantly populate most urban areas from different areas, and relative anonymity blurs the caste lines. However, because of the temporal and spatial continuity, rural areas persist in beliefs related to purity and pollution drawn from the caste system, adversely affecting sanitation. Therefore, intervention in sanitation involves changing notions of purity and pollution related to caste hierarchy.

The National Annual Rural Sanitation Survey (NARSS) data indicates that 77% of households have access to toilets, of which 93.4% use them regularly. The survey also suggests that 95.6% of the ODF-verified villages have been confirmed as ODF and 70% had the least litter and stagnant water ((Ministry of Drinking Water and Sanitation (u.d.) According to the World Bank, from 2011 to 2015, despite having a higher GDP, India had the lowest share of the population with improved sanitation compared to Bangladesh, Pakistan, Vietnam, and Sri Lanka. The evidence shows that poverty may not be the only cause of inadequate sanitation coverage in India. Embedded factors, including culture, social norms, behaviour, and institutions, are additional factors that may be responsible for the coverage and use of improved sanitation.

Intervention Programmes

The successive governments in India launched several sanitation programmes, viz. the Central Rural Sanitation Programme (CRSP) in 1986 and the TSC in 1999. More recently, the central government initiated the Swachh Bharat Mission (Gramin) (SBM(G)) as a submission under the Swachh Bharat Mission on 2 October 2014. The mission aimed at improving villages' cleanliness by managing solid and liquid waste combined with the thrust on open defecation-free (ODF) villages (vide Joint Secretary's DO letter dated 9 June 2015).

> ODF is the termination of faecal-oral transmission, defined by a) no visible faeces found in the environment/village, and b) every household and public/community institutions using safe technology option for disposal of faeces.

The planning for implementing the mission is done at the district level, focusing on collective behaviour change at the village level through awareness generation and triggering desirable action. These activities are intended to generate awareness and trigger demand for toilets. They are labelled as information, education, and communication (IEC) activities. IEC activities are at the heart of any behaviour change programme, which provides knowledge about the dangers of continuing with the existing behaviour (open defecation) and the benefits that the individuals and community will have by adopting the advocated behaviour (construction and use of toilets). Secondly, to propel individuals and communities to action, the IEC strategy links its activities to the message's underlying sociocultural and emotional aspects. IEC activities are most important for collective behaviour change through interpersonal communication (IPC) and door-to-door contact. Village-level motivators, known as 'Swachhata Doot', would facilitate these activities. The literal translation would be ambassadors of cleanliness or sanitation messengers and non-governmental agencies (NGOs). Technology and media are also essential elements of overall communication strategy. The IEC activities would be planned according to the recommendations and advice of Rapid Action Learning Units (RALUs) constituted at national, state, and district levels for studying and analysing the programme implementation.

The activities under IEC involved interpersonal communication, which involved *Swachhata Doot* reaching the household, appraising the importance of the construction of toilets, and discussing various dangers related to open defecation. They also used ambient media like graffiti in schools, public toilets, and other public places to reach their audience. The government used mass media like radio programmes, television advertisements, and print media to reach a larger audience. The Swachh Bharat logo (a symbolic representation of Gandhi) became ubiquitous, ranging from railway platforms to currency notes. The effort was gigantic because it intended to touch one-sixth of humanity with a low literacy rate and change habits and cultural nuances that have existed for thousands of years. A report on assessing the reach and value of IEC activities under the Swachh Bharat Mission (Gramin – Ministry of Drinking Water and Sanitation, 2019) estimated that an average rural person was exposed to IEC about 2500–3000 times from 2014 to 2019. The report estimated that interpersonal communication (IPC) accounted for 50% of the communication mix among the methods adopted. The report observed that the recall value of IPC was much higher than any other channels used.

The IEC was followed by capacity building, availability of sanitation materials, and construction of individual household toilets. Since 2 October 2014, 19.07 million toilets have been constructed, accounting for a 10.52% increase in the availability of toilets in households. More than 63000 villages have been declared ODF. Against the target of 5 million individual toilets for households (2014–15), about 5.8 million toilets were constructed. Additionally, more than 1100 community sanitary complexes were constructed. More than 25000 school toilets and over 8000 Anganwadi toilets were constructed for students. More importantly, about five million household toilets were constructed after SBM (G) launch. Thus, during the post-SBM (G) period, there was a considerable acceleration in the pace of toilet construction compared to the pre-SBM period (National Statistical Commission Annual Report, 2016–17). However, sanitation coverage is as dispersed as the states' geographical positions and socio-economic dynamics. The coverage is as low as 25% in Bihar and 96% in Kerala. Madhya Pradesh and Andhra Pradesh are placed around the middle, with 45% coverage. Gujarat and West Bengal have around 75% coverage. As per the NSSO 2015 survey, Sikkim received the first rank on sanitation parameters, while Telangana was placed 13th in the ranking list.

Similarly, Gujarat and Bihar received 14th and 21st positions, respectively. As per the report, 61.1% of Telangana households have sanitary toilets, and 97.8% have access to toilets and use them. 55.5% and 31.6% of households in Gujarat and Bihar had sanitary toilets, respectively. Furthermore, 96.2% and 94.2% of households with sanitary toilets in Gujarat and Bihar had access to toilets and used them, respectively. The coverage dispersion depicts diverse preferences for sanitation and affordability of toilets across regions. The National Annual Rural Sanitation Survey (NARSS) 2017–18 found that about 77% of the households had access to toilets. In all these, one can see that the programme's progress is primarily measured by the construction of toilets and the villages' ODF status.

Swachh Bharat Mission (Gramin)

In contrast, the primary objective of SBM(G) is behaviour change which leads to households realising the importance of toilets for better physical and mental health for all family members and generating demand for the construction and use of toilets. The focus shifting to the construction of toilets is easy to understand. The number of toilets constructed is far easier to count and monitor than to monitor and quantitatively capture behaviour change at the individual and household levels. There is hardly any study measuring the extent of behaviour change achieved during the programme. Moreover, there has not been any evaluation of the actual implementation of the different IEC activities and their impact on household sanitation behaviour. In a meeting of government officials, it was indicated that there is a lack of information on factors that drive household decisions towards toilet construction.[1] IEC activities are likely to motivate people to construct a toilet. Toilet construction under SBM(G) would also depend on the toilet design, supply of sanitation materials on time, and the political and social leadership. O'Reilly and Louis (2014) found that successful sanitation adoption depends on the government's multi-scalar political will and NGOs' involvement. However, reliable water supply, compatible soil type, and changing land use provide the facilitative ecosystem for constructing and using toilets.

There are a few challenges in front of SBM(G). Social conformity delays the change process. When children and other family members observe their family, friends, and other community members defecate in the open, they perceive it as a social norm – a behavioural rule that most people prefer to conform because they believe that most people in the community conform and they should also conform (Bicchieri 2016). Thus, it gets rooted in the culture. Thus, it is perceived as a part of behaviour rooted in the local culture. It is a traditional practice and part of one's daily routine. They also see it as part of their socialisation norms and habits. One of the significant departures of SBM(G) from the earlier programmes is to focus on the whole Gram Panchayat (GP) rather than the social groups. Its focus is community-level behaviour change, which is somewhat fragmented and often riddled with conflicts. Collective behaviour change of the GP is more accessible when the whole GP is homogeneous. Empirical evidence reveals that open defecation is higher in the village with more conflicts (Hathi et al., 2016).

As sanitation combines private behaviours with most public impact (McGranahan, 2015), the challenge of collective action may lead to failure to provide a clean public good environment. Co-production of a clean environment with the government's support may hinder collective decision-making if political brokerage manipulates the distribution of benefits for political advantage (McGranahan, 2015). Furthermore, pit toilet construction poses a typical challenge within a caste-based hierarchical society. Pit toilets get filled up in a few years and need emptying. However, the notions of caste-based purity and pollution prevent the upper-caste households from constructing toilets as they will not empty them. They will depend on other caste people to come and do the 'dirty' job of cleaning the pits. Thus, constructing pit toilets in certain areas poses sociocultural challenges that must be overcome. The cultural norms regarding human waste may create barriers to developing an appropriate and cost-effective excreta management system (Jewitt, 2011).

Because of the construction design and structure of the toilets (lack of ventilation and natural light), many villagers report that they found closed toilets repulsive. Most rural households cannot afford cleaning agents to keep toilets clean and free of foul smells. Thus, the image that toilets are smelly, dark, small, enclosed spaces that need to be avoided has become deep-rooted in the minds of rural people. As a result of this perception, many choose not to use closed toilets and often express that they derive more comfort from defecating in the open air. They also associate open defecation with the health benefits of clean air. In 2014, before SBM(G) started, 140000 deaths occurred due to diarrhoeal disease attributed to unsafe sanitation. It was also reported that before implementing SBM(G), the total death due to diarrhoea was about 450000, out of which about 39000 were children below five years of age (Swachh Bharat Mission – Preliminary estimations of potential health impacts from increased sanitation coverage, 2019). The demand for toilets for better health outcomes is also questionable as evidence of the impact of the toilet on sanitation behaviour and health outcomes is mixed. A randomised control trial conducted in rural Madhya Pradesh to analyse the impact of the Total Sanitation Campaign (TSC) on defecation behaviour and child health reveals that the intervention led to a modest increase in household toilet use. These improvements were insufficient for better child health outcomes (Patil et al., 2014). However, another randomised control trial conducted in rural Orissa reveals that the sanitation campaign increases toilet use and positively impacts child health (Dickinson et al., 2015). Therefore, the impact of the sanitation campaign is context-specific. The drivers of a successful campaign need to be understood in a broader context. The drivers from the demand side could be expected health outcomes, personal cleanliness, convenience, privacy, and affordability. The supply-side drivers could be the availability of trained human resources and construction materials.

This book analyses the factors contributing to toilet use at the household level. In other words, we wanted to identify factors that would lead to adopting toilets among people who have been using open spaces for defecation. It is estimated that in India alone, more than 65000 children could be saved annually by improving water sanitation and hygiene; therefore, it is also critical to analyse factors that would reduce open defecation. One of the significant arguments that has been advocated earlier is that lack of toilets is the cause of open defecation. However, earlier research suggests that despite having constructed toilets people have not been using them because of various other factors. It is well acknowledged that toilet interventions should not be just about constructing toilets. It has to go beyond and explore psychological, sociocultural, and economic factors that will lead to toilet adoption (O'Riley & Louis, 2014) because toilet use requires a change of habits. Habits are zones of comfort for the individual. Western societies, mainly because of climatic conditions, had to adjust to defecating in a closed place even though early closed toilets were smelly and dirty. With time, the users of the closed toilets also devised ways to keep them clean and less smelly. However, rain is intermittent in India, where most of the year is sunny. With low population density, open defecation was accepted as a norm rather than an exception. Thus, the habits that have been formed and have become part of the sociocultural milieu needed a large-scale programme for changing social norms and behaviour. To fully appreciate the reasons behind the success or failure of any intervention programme, we need to discuss the profound implications of open defecation for individuals, communities, and nations.

Further, this book attempts to identify and analyse the factors embedded in the cultural practices, the construction and structural aspects of toilets, and individual-level habits that act as barriers to adopting toilets in rural households. Often, adopting a new behaviour implies fully or partially replacing existing behaviour entailing individuals and communities to move from their comfort zones. Transitioning to a new behaviour entails associated perceived risks. However, individuals and communities must adopt new behaviour for advancement and well-being. The new behaviour may include smoking cessation to the adoption of flush toilets. Individuals frequently make cost-benefit analyses in decision-making using available heuristics. The cost and benefits are not always financial or quantifiable; they are often abstract and qualitative. For example, 'shame' is a cost paid for open defecation. The cost here is expressed in terms of the discomfort experienced by the person. The benefit of a flush toilet may be 'security' for the person. When the perceived risk in the advocated behaviour (adoption of toilets) is lower than the perceived risks in the existing behaviour (open defecation), people are more likely to adopt the behaviour. However, many variables intervene in increasing or decreasing a particular behaviour's perceived costs or benefits. Reviewing existing literature, secondary data, and primary research, we attempt to understand the perceived risks in existing behaviour (open defecation) and the advocated behaviour (using toilets). We also try to identify the elements in information, education, and communication (IEC) found effective or ineffective under different conditions. We attempt to understand the relative effectiveness of the communication mix (emotion-heavy and fact-heavy content) and message framing (gain framing and loss framing) for toilet construction and behaviour change. This book attempts to unravel how cultural aspects play a role and how social inequality of gender and caste and political brokerage affect toilet construction and its uses. It also analyses the supply-side bottlenecks, the effect of reliable water supply, and the changes in land use affecting the readiness to construct toilets.

Note

1 Consultative workshop on forward planning of Rapid Action Learning Units (RAULs) in states to support SBM(G) in Lucknow on 23 June 2016.

2 Sanitation Policies, Programmes, and Actions

Historical Background

A toilet within the residence is commonly believed to be a Western innovation. Western societies' preponderance of toilets within the house is primarily attributed to the harsh climatic conditions. Because of the inclement weather in the temperate zones, people would have preferred to have toilets within their houses. In a hot country with milder weather conditions, people would have preferred to go outside to defecate in the open rather than stay within the closed environment of the home. However, these arguments are belied by the fact that in Harappa Mohenjo-Daro (part of the Indus Valley Civilisation), almost every house had a private bath and toilet area with drains to take dirty water into the larger cesspool dating to the mid-third millennium. In ancient India, sanitation was a core component of daily rituals; a detailed description is found in *Manusmriti* (Tiwary & Saurabh, 2018). Indus Valley was known for excellent sanitation facilities, substantiated by the remnants of toilets that have been found in the historical sites of Mohenjo-Daro and Harappa (Khan, 2014). However, with the onset of colonial rule in the subcontinent, sanitation ceased to be a priority. Gradual marginalisation of the natives increased rural poverty under British colonial rule; the rise of urban spaces, population growth, and general apathy of administration were critical reasons sanitation lost priority.

In 1859 British troops recorded a high mortality rate in India because of the spread of diarrhoea. The government took notice of the sanitation situation, and the Commission for Public Health was set up. Subsequently, under the Military Cantonments Act of 1865, sanitary boards were established to administer the sanitation conditions for the civilian population. However, the focus of the colonial government remained centred around the European civilian population in different cities, often referred to as civil lines in northern Indian towns and the cantonment areas. Most of the 'native' parts of the towns lacked civic amenities. In addition, most of the municipal reforms during that time focused on eradicating epidemics and constructing estates but did not address the sanitation needs of the Indians. Despite the population being manageable, public health and sanitation were never prioritised (Halvorson and Wescoat 2020; Ramasubban 2008).

Instead of trying to intervene and bring sanitation to the forefront, the colonial government had overlooked the sanitation needs of Indians and taken advantage of

DOI: 10.4324/9781032726267-2

the existing caste divide that made the lowest rung in the social hierarchy the manual scavengers to do the dirty jobs. All cantonments and the civil lines (for British and European populations) employed manual scavengers. It not only maintained the existing caste-related power hierarchy but also strengthened the dominant views of pollution and purity that also kept the manual scavenging going. Mahatma Gandhi did not accept the division of society and the inhuman nature of manual scavenging. Gandhi spearheaded a movement against the disgrace of untouchability. His fight against manual scavenging might have distanced him from his near and dear ones for some time. Still, his efforts led to establishing the Harijan Sevak Sangh in 1932 for the manual scavengers, which was instrumental in launching sanitation awareness. Joshi and Khattri (2019) have succulently, as put it.

> For Gandhi, withering away of the caste-based inequalities were essential for achieving a state of complete health, well-being, cleanliness and freedom. The notion of swaraj for Gandhi is intricately linked to the issue of cleanliness and sanitation.
>
> (Joshi & Khattri, 2019, pp. 3–4)

Sanitation: Post-Independence Scenario

In 1950, water supply and sanitation became part of the health sector. However, the major thrust to sanitation came with the United Nations's (UN's) call for access to safe drinking water and adequate sanitation facility for all, and it initiated the International Drinking Water Supply and Sanitation Decade (1981–90). Launched in 1981, it targeted 25% toilet coverage in rural India. In 1990, sanitation coverage extended to a measly number of 2.45% from 0.50% recorded at the beginning of the decade. Thus, as O'Rourke (1992) had pointed out worldwide, the International Drinking Water Supply and Sanitation Decade (1981–90) was a significant failure. There was nothing to talk about the decade as it had squandered an excellent opportunity to make the country defecation free.

The year 1986 was a turning point in the history of rural sanitation. That year, rural sanitation was shifted to the Ministry of Rural Development (MoRD) and the nationwide sanitation programme's planning, implementation, supervising, and coordination (GoI, 2002). Simultaneously, the Council for Advancement of People's Action and Rural Technology (CAPART) was formed in the same year. One of the critical areas entrusted to CAPART was to hasten the implementation of rural sanitation programmes leveraging its network of local-level non-governmental organisations (Chaudhary, n.d.). Thus, the Central Rural Sanitation Programme (CRSP), operational from 1986 to 1999, was the first structured programme launched by the MoRD. However, its progress was slow due to lack of awareness and lower adoption and did not automatically translate into usage. From 1996 to 1997, a survey by the Indian Institute of Mass Communication reported that most people (55%) of households with a toilet at home were self-motivated to use it. A majority of the users reported that they used the toilet because of convenience and privacy. In the study, 51% of the respondents were ready to spend Rs 1000 to have a toilet at home. Based on these findings, the CRSP moved from a top-down approach to a demand-driven one.

Consequently, thirteen years later, the central government launched the Total Sanitation Campaign (TSC) in 1999 by decentralised planning and implementation through village panchayats, focusing on demand-based toilet construction. In 2003, Nirmal Gram Puraskar (NGP) was set up and financially rewarded to the Gram Panchayats for attaining 100% sanitation. Almost a decade later, the Ministry of Rural Development launched the National Urban Sanitation Policy (NUSP) with the lofty vision of universal sanitation coverage and open defecation-free cities in India (GoI, u.d.). With the success of NGP, the Total Sanitation Campaign (TSC) was renamed Nirmal Bharat Abhiyan (NBA) in 2012. It facilitated the installation of toilets in below-poverty-line (BPL) households and government institutions in villages.

The Total Sanitation Campaign (1999–2011) marked a change in India's sanitation policy to achieve universal rural sanitation coverage by 2012 through social mobilisations and Information, Education and Communication (IEC) activities. The Total Sanitation Campaign, afterwards re-christened as Nirmal Bharat Abhiyan (2012–14), aimed at improving the quality of life in terms of health and well-being by accelerating the rate coverage of rural households in terms of construction and use of toilets; it focused on rural areas with new strategies and techniques to achieve its objectives by 2022. This campaign covered all rural households with the financial assistance to construct toilets was extended to all the below poverty line (BPL) and above poverty line (APL) households. With the change in the government at the centre in 2014, the Nirmal Bharat Abhiyan (NBA) was modified substantially and was launched as Swachh Bharat Abhiyan (SBM). The SBM was targeted at achieving universal sanitation coverage within four years. The first three sanitation programs (CRSP, TSC, and NBA) only catered to the rural population's sanitation needs. In contrast, SBM was aimed at both rural and urban populations. Thus, it had two sub-missions, the Swachh Bharat Mission (Gramin) and the Swachh Bharat Mission (Urban).

Issues Emerging in Construction and Usage of Toilets

One central question that has been doing the rounds in the policy domain of sanitation is whether the successive sanitation programmes were conceived as stage improvements over the previous ones or brought about a paradigm change in how the original programmes were conceived. In this context, it is crucial to understand the impacts of these sanitation programmes on individuals, households, and the community. Thus, a literature review of studies on these campaigns and explicitly addressing these aspects was carried out. Following the launch of various sanitation programmes by each successive government (before SBM), in 2005, the Department of Drinking Water Supply of the MoRD was commissioned to conduct a mid-term evaluation of TSC in 14 states to assess its efficiency and effectiveness. It was found that the adoption rate of toilets has increased, but the lack of sanitation facilities has been one of the main issues in the campaign. The study report found that clogging of toilets, the small size of toilets, and lack of water were the chief reasons for members of the households not using their toilets.

Further, poor households' lack of space within the home has been a significant deterrent in constructing toilets, along with the cultural factor that has been a significant obstacle. For example, while women preferred toilets at home for safety and dignity, the elderly male members would object to it. Thus, many households suffered from a lack of consensus and did not adopt toilets. Another non-structural reason for not having a toilet at home was the lack of money for constructing toilets. In a similar tune, later studies also echoed the previous findings. They stated that the habit of open defecation and its attendant rituals posed a significant threat to using toilets at home and conforming to the overall state of sanitation within the village (Banda et al., 2007).

In 2008, WaterAid India studied the factors that facilitated toilet adoption and acted as barriers to toilet adoption during the Total Sanitation Campaign (TSC) period. The analysis of the study results suggested that TSC suffered from the top-down implementation approach. The government-led programme had become target driven and deviated from the envisaged people-centric approach. Toilet coverage was uneven across states and districts. The target group's preferences were not considered, and innovations in toilet design and the use of technology in water management were neglected. The study indicated that TSC was poorly implemented and failed to translate the policy into action. The study also reported that most local government representatives or PRI functionaries were unaware of the TSC and its roles until the *Nirmal Gram Puraskar*s were awarded. During the same year, another assessment study of TSC conducted by WaterAid India found specific innovations in the information, education, and communication sectors that led to a competitive spirit, active participation and partnerships of the target group members, and the involvement of women. The study noted that rural sanitary markets or production centres were absent in many places, women's sanitary complexes were poorly maintained, and there were no monitoring and follow-up measures.

Using a cluster randomised design, Pattanayak et al. (2009) examined the shame versus subsidy debate effects in two blocks of Bhadrak District in Odisha. There has been a raging debate among researchers and policymakers about the relative importance of subsidy in adopting toilets over shaming – creating strong intrinsic motivation by paying for the services. The study found that the adopted information, education, and communication strategies had successfully moved people from open defecation to using toilets at home. It had a substantial impact on toilet adoption. Several exciting points emerged from the study. Awareness that open defecation causes diarrhoea did not translate to using toilets. Rather issues of privacy and dignity of women were the key influencing factors in adopting toilets. Secondly, the information, education, and communication campaigns targeted communities rather than individuals, creating social pressures to conform because the information had permeated widely in the community and helped overcome individual-level passivity. During the same year, research investigating the sanitation status in

India suggested that various sociocultural, geographic, and economic differentials blocked access to universal sanitation despite the enormity of the situation and the need for toilets on a large scale. The powerful caste-based differences often mire sanitation coverage. Further analysis found differences in the resistance to toilets that certain areas and population groups had greater resistance to adopting household sanitation facilities than others. After the decade of TSC, World Bank-WSP's (2010) assessment of the Total Sanitation Campaign suggested that the basic principles of the Total Sanitation Campaign were not adhered to in more than 50% of the sampled villages (Bonu and Kim 2009).

In a cross-sectional study of the Total Sanitation Campaign (TSC) during 2012 in Odisha, it was reported that during the period, the toilet coverage in the 20 villages understudy had gone up drastically. The study found that the non-usage of toilets was due to inconvenience and incomplete construction of toilets. Many villagers had converted the toilets into storerooms. Other reasons for non-use were toilets lacking privacy, being broken, or being blocked (Barnard et al., 2013). A study by the Planning Commission (2013) evaluated the TSC to assess its impact on the quality of life, mainly on the rural poor, and the durability of sanitation facilities. The study reported that the principal reasons for OD practice were lack of awareness (IEC), established age-old practices, and the non-availability of adequate water for toilet use, consistent with 2010 WSP's evaluation. Another study in 2013 explored the causes of the gaps in the policy and practice of TSC. The study was conducted in Uttar Pradesh, Madhya Pradesh, Haryana, and Himachal Pradesh. The data analysis suggested similar findings to the World Bank-WSP report, as there was a mismatch between the principles of TSC and their implementation. Like many other earlier evaluations of TSC, they concluded that the TSC was government led, infrastructure centred, subsidy based, and supply led, which is consistent with earlier evaluations of the TSC's poor outcomes. However, the study found rare household motivation and involvement in toilet construction. Flawed monitoring was an additional shortcoming of the TSC.

A survey found that government-constructed toilets were less likely to be used than privately built toilets (Coffey et al., 2014). It further predicted that the toilets would remain unused if constructed without changing the target group's preferences. In another study, the impact of TSC on the availability of toilets was assessed; it was found that 19% of villages reported the availability of improved sanitation facilities. However, the intervention did not improve the child's health, measured using different health outcomes. Despite a modest increase in the number of toilets, there was no improvement in different child health parameters. It became clear that universal coverage is essential for better child health outcomes. Even if only a handful of people in the village practice open defecation, it can contaminate the water sources and become the harbinger of ill health. It inferred that the treatment and intervention were insufficient to improve child health outcomes though there were modest increases in the number of Individual Household Latrines (IHLs). On the contrary, a randomised control trial conducted in rural Orissa revealed that the sanitation campaigns increase the use of toilets and positively impact child health (Dickinson et al., 2015).

Sociocultural and Behavioural Aspects

Sociocultural factors impact sanitation behaviour as much as economic factors on access and use of toilets (De, 2018). These non-economic factors include gender, age, education of the household head, and the number of household members. Regional effects impact access to sanitation, implying norms and customs impacting sanitation. Quality, cleanliness, and other personal preferences matter in the use of toilets. The issue of cleanliness has a social-cultural and behavioural dimension; Speltini and Passini (2014) point out that fear of getting contaminated and cleaning practices are rooted in cultural practices. Specifically, there is a connection between one's sense of cleanliness and attitudes of prejudice and intolerance towards others. Dittmer (2009), in problematising the issue of abandoning the practice of open defecation, believed that it was always not linked to the presence or absence of water or toilets but 'social determinants' and social convention reinforced by traditional beliefs. Dittmer (2009) identifies beliefs as social and cultural barriers to adopting improved sanitation. However, the author found a possible way of encouraging social change and engaging with communities to end open defecation by mapping social communication channels relevant to each community. Coffey and Spears (2017) observed that poverty is not the only contributor to open defecation; it is bolstered by the caste system, including untouchability and purity rituals. They write that increased funding and ever more new toilets are critical and timely calls for destroying the social barriers for the fundamental shift in policy perspectives to effect a crucial, much overdue change. Similarly, Vyas's (2018) study also pointed out that the open defecation practice is related to 'rituals of purity and pollution that discourage having toilets close to house'.

Investigating the impact of sociocultural and behavioural aspects on toilets and sanitation practices in the household, Routray et al. (2017) provided the reasons for lower adoption, especially the government's subsidised toilets. This study revealed that cultural practices affected toilet adoption and use, resulting in rituals that reinforce certain habits restricting handling and containing adult human faeces near homes. The study further pointed out that lack of capacity and skills among people at the operational level negatively impacted the implementation of sanitation campaigns. Further, power hierarchies and intergenerational and household dynamics in household decisions, including toilet installation, were additional reasons for the non-adoption of toilets in the household. Sociocultural practices profoundly affect the population's health, affecting the healthcare delivery system (Wasonga et al., 2016). Jenkins and Curtis (2005) pointed out that health considerations played a minor role and had little impact on preventing faecal-oral disease transmission. To achieve the total sanitation goal, Waterkeyn and Cairncross (2005) opine that by altering the norms of a community, a culture of cleanliness and hygienic behaviour can be improved that directs behaviour towards more effective control of family health.

Jenkins and Scott (2007) point out that adopting improved toilets depends on developing specific preferences. It results from the dissatisfaction arising out of existing practices and is supported by awareness and availability of alternatives to overcome the present state of sanitation. They maintained that the households go through several stages before finally adopting toilets. In the beginning, the households start planning for sanitation change. However, all households are not at the same level in the planning process. Some of the factors are within the control of the households (e.g. handwashing, cleaning, etc.). Some, like the infrastructure for sanitation, are outside the control of the households because of a lack of resources. Various psychological factors affect the readiness to adopt toilets which have been largely ignored in the discourse on adopting toilets. The natural reaction of human beings to excreta is disgust. Therefore, open defecation in high OD density areas is likely to generate disgust and likelihood of adoption will be high whenever the opportunity for a flush/pour toilet arises. In an exciting study on narratives of sanitation, Leong (2020) came across a paradoxical situation where despite all the information, education, communication initiatives and the availability of money to construct toilets, people have consistently shown a preference for open defecation.

Deacon and Olatunjib's (2007) study indicated that disgust sensitivity was positively related to anxious and avoidant responses to the contamination-related fear. The findings indicate that disgust sensitivity has a specific strong relationship with concerns for contamination, usually found among patients suffering from obsessive-compulsive disorder in a disease avoidance model. Schnall et al. (2008) found cognitive cleanliness uniquely reduced the severity of moral judgement by removing the feeling of disgust. On the other hand, physical cleanliness was instrumental in reducing the intensity of moral judgement only when considered along with cognitive cleanliness.

The Merger of Techno-Cultural Factors

Most sanitation efforts have looked at the technological, cultural, and structural factors separately. However, there have been attempts to integrate. However, such initiatives got stuck at the planning stage, and there was no relationship between the integrative approach at the planning stage and the implementation at the ground level. Therefore, to solve the global challenge of sanitation Van Vliet et al. (2010) observed that to be effective, sanitation programmes should be designed to fit within the physical and societal systems. Seetharam (2015) suggested a framework for assessing the technological aspects of sanitation. He proposed that sanitation be viewed as an integrated value chain process and should be internalised by all actors. Kaliski (2015) offered an economic model of human behaviour and political ecology approaches to understand the factors that can increase or decrease an individual's demand for toilet construction and sanitation. Her study investigates sanitation from an economic, political, cultural, or historical framework and tries to understand the origins of public health problems and complications in preventing the demand for toilets. In an overall observation of the adaptation and changes in sanitation practices, Fagbemiro et al. (2016) opine that the effective utilisation of sanitation information depends on social structures, education, cultural beliefs and practices, and economic, government, and environmental conditions. O'Reilly and Louis (2014) argue that the construction of toilets is significant and getting people to use them is crucial for public health. However, it depends on three factors; they are labelled as the toilet tripod. The first leg of the tripod is the political will meaning the will to govern. The campaign becomes effective when the local government is proactive and supported with resources from the central government programmes. The second leg of the tripod is the proximate social pressure and economic change. They found that economic growth, increasing household income, and exposure to urban lifestyles made people adopt toilets readily. The third leg of the tripod was the political ecology supported by state investments. For example, increasing population density made it difficult for people to defecate in open spaces. It was also found that better access to drinking water was critical in adopting toilets. Thus, macroeconomic factors, drinking water availability, population density, state investments, and soil conditions contribute to adopting toilets (O'Reilly & Louis, 2014). However, the context chosen by O'Reilly and Louis was two states, focusing on political and economic factors rather than the cultural ones.

The collective behaviour of the community could be one of the most critical determinants of successful sanitation. As sanitation combines personal behaviours with the most significant public impact (McGranahan, 2015), the challenge of collective action could lead to failure to provide a clean environment that is a public good. The cultural norms regarding human waste may create barriers to developing appropriate and cost-effective excreta management systems (Jewitt, 2011). Wherever pit toilets are constructed, it becomes necessary to empty the pit after a few years. Depending on the size of the pit and usage, the pit may get filled between two to five years. Because of the caste hierarchy and the notion of pollution and purity, most people would not like to clear the pit, so the toilet becomes unusable. It takes time for people to change their mindset to distinguish between ritualistic pollution and actual pollution, which is unhealthy. Once they can traverse this space, they can also transform it into an attached bathroom at home (see Srinivas, 2002). Collective behavioural change becomes more manageable when the entire village or community is homogeneous. Empirical evidence reveals that open defecation is higher in villages with more conflicts (Hathi et al., 2016).

Sanitation is a comprehensive intervention that promotes sanitation behaviours and creates access to cleanliness, safe water, toilets, drainage facilities, waste management, and water treatment facilities. Implementing sanitation activities requires community participation, government contribution in policy level and budget allocation, indigenous resources, and local practices. India is the second largest populated country with more than 138 crores of population. As per the population growth demand providing access to sanitation is a significant challenge for the country. Sanitation impacts India's health burden and GDP, as due to lack of proper sanitation the major waterborne diseases like diarrhoea, malaria, typhoid, and hepatitis are creating significant damage to public health. The Government of India has been legislating various policies and schemes to create sanitation services, i.e., water treatment, sewerage management, human wastage management, and solid and liquid waste management. The lack of sanitation facilities for rural masses is not entirely due to low income. Still, many other factors, including behaviour, gender, caste, education, and general living standards like housing quality, wealth, and material comfort of people, determine their preference for sanitation. People's preference for sanitation may trail behind the preference for several other essential amenities like *pakka* house, electricity, water connection, etc.

On the other hand, social norms of purity may discourage households from constructing toilets inside the house or even within the premises. Avoiding toilets may worsen if the construction quality is not up to the mark or the structure is inconvenient for use. The lack of adequate water supply may make the situation worse. Hence there is a need to design less water-using toilets for the water crisis-facing states like Rajasthan, Gujarat, Jharkhand, Andhra Pradesh, and Karnataka. The implementation mechanism is not always efficient, and many operational challenges emerge at the national, state, and community levels. Information, education, and communication (IEC), including outreach strategies and having accredited the services of SBM volunteers, has been ineffective in generating demand for toilets. An institutional mechanism with a proper incentive structure to discourage open defecation is mostly not in place. The Swachh Baharat Abhiyan has introduced a subsidy of Rs 12000 for toilet construction and encouraged volunteerism by conducting summer internship programmes with a cash prize ranging from Rs 10000 to Rs 100000. The other incentive schemes like the Nirmal Bharat Abhiyan offer Rs 50000 to Rs 1000000 incentives for each Open Defecation free (ODF) declared Gram Panchayats.

Income along with higher expenditure on durable goods impacts uptake of sanitation. The sanitation programme is more likely to succeed in Sikkim, Kerala, Mizoram, and Nagaland where employment and income-generation programmes are delivered efficiently. The Ministry of Housing and Urban Affairs (MoHUA) has initiated a collaboration between the National Urban Livelihoods Mission (NULM) and the Swachh Bharat Mission (SBM). It has entrusted the operation and maintenance of public and community toilets contract to Urban SHG groups which consist of a minimum of 10% of sanitation workers or other ultra poor members. An aspirational household with increasing income and living standards is likelier to build and use the toilet. The household toilets and sanitation behaviours will increase family health, self-respect, safety, and security. Many diseases arise from houseflies and mosquitos, and water and food contamination will decrease due to toilet usage. As a result, the household expenditures on health problems will be reduced, and every family member will lead a healthy and prosperous life. There is a need to create income generation for local bodies or SHG members in handholding and assigning the maintenance of community toilet facilities, potable water systems, sewerage, and solid and liquid waste management for the programme's long-term sustainability. Hence, sanitation programmes may converge with other employment generation or livelihood programmes. The sanitation programme is more likely to be successful in regions where population density is higher, viz. Indore, Surat, Vijayawada, Mumbai, Pune, Raipur, Bhopal, Vadodara, Visakhapatnam, Ahmedabad, etc. Due to the density of population spaces, open defecation is not generally available. Hence, the implementation authorities may target areas where the population density is higher or urbanisation is gradually occurring.

The Information, Education, and Communication (IEC)

The successful implementation of the sanitation programme depends upon the effectiveness of the IEC also, as the sanitation intervention aims to change the community's attitudes on open defecation, cleanliness, drainage system, waste management, etc. Information, education, and communication (IEC) attempts to motivate a target audience concerning specific problems, particularly in preventive healthcare, by providing knowledge about the causative factors of specific health problems and how they can be alleviated by adopting specific alternative behaviour and practices. Research has pointed out that IEC has created awareness and knowledge and resulted in behaviour change (World Health Organization, 2001). Through IEC and the use of mass media, many taboo subjects may come within the ambit of public debate and slowly make the idea of change a point of conversation (Cofie et al., 2013). However, the IEC may fail without interpersonal communication and creating word of mouth through local-level influencers. The IEC can efficiently sensitise the target population irrespective of age, gender, and literacy levels. It educates the community on the adverse effects of lack of sanitisation, and the importance of sanitation enhances the knowledge levels and role clarity and promotes sanitation behaviours. The Government of India has spent an amount of 1894.85 crores for IEC material under Swachh Bharat Mission (G) from 2014–15 to 2021–2.

Social Behaviour Change Communication (SBCC)

One of the significant drawbacks of IEC is that it is one-way communication. Experts often prepare the IEC materials, and the target group is often 'bombarded' with the information they cannot relate to or think is unimplementable. Because of its one-way nature, it cannot engage the target audience and thus lacks the motivational thrust. On the other hand, Social and Behaviour Change Communication (SBCC) is an effective strategy to promote sanitation behaviour among the target population (Mckee et al., 2014). As changes in sanitation, behaviour requires comprehensive intervention that includes hygiene, water management, waste management, sewerage management, and promotion of individual and community toilets. Each requires community participation as a mandatory element. It needs community engagement. Mainly, the individuals and household members need to be sensitised on the importance of sanitation, its effects on public health, increased health burden, and the consequence of inclusive growth. The SBCC strategy includes applying participative rural appraisal (PRA) tools, developing relevant communication materials, and carrying out mid-media activities. The mid-media activities like cultural programmes, competitions, debates, poster making, street shows, *Kala Jathas*, wall writings, rallies, etc. are helpful to reach the expected outcomes.

Sanitation in Aspirational Districts

The Government of India initiated the 'Transformation of Aspirational District Program' in 2018 to improve the living standards of the districts located in remote, undeveloped, neglected, and left-wing extremism areas. A total of 2778 villages from 117 districts were selected for this project. Sanitation is a critical determinant in improving living standards and promoting self-sustained solid and liquid waste management systems for selected aspirational districts.

Community-Level Workers. The role of community-level workers like AWW, ANM, ASHA, and postal service employees is essential for rendering comprehensive sanitation. For this purpose, the Swachh Bharat Gramin scheme has introduced the *Swachhagrahis* position on incentivised payment basis in selected villages. The Swachhagrahis would promote behaviour changes among community members and sustain sanitation behaviour. They should be trained on different aspects of behaviour change communication. They should also be trained in using the PRA tools (triggering) to work effectively in the community. The Swachhagrahis conduct early morning visits to common open defecation (OD) places under the *Nigrani* strategy. The objective of these visits is to sensitise the community to stop open defecation.

Design of the Toilets

Given challenges in reaching 100% ODF, the design of the toilets may be re-examined to meet the aspiration of the households, such as comfortability in usage, low-cost construction, and minimal place and water consumption. The following cost-effective designs have been introduced as part of rural sanitation.

Twin Pit Toilets. The design of the twin pit toilet comprises two substitute pits with three feet of depth and connects to a pour flush toilet. The water released from toilets falls in one pit and penetrates the soil; the faecal matter will be removable. The twin pit technology has advantages like comparatively low-cost construction between Rs 12000 and 15000; minimal water requirement, about one and a half to two litres per usage; faecal matter conversion into manure; and non-requirement of manual scavengers. But the major bottleneck is the perception of people. They think the twin pits of around three feet are too small and would get filled very soon. Households perceive the removal of sludge from filled pits as problematic. There is fear of groundwater contamination in the twin pit model due to high-groundwater level, and flooding. However, percolation chances in rocky soil is negligible. Furthermore, in the twin-pit model the toilet room or superstructure is relatively narrow and causes inconvenience. The non-availability of a preferred place per belief on Vasthu is one of the other constraints for constructing the twin pit toilets.

Eco-San Toilets. The eco-san toilets are developed for water scarcity areas. These toilets are constructed above the land level and have two chambers, including three separate chambers to collect urine, water, and faecal matter. The construction cost of an eco-san toilet varies between Rs 16000 to Rs 22000, which is prohibitively high for people in rural areas. Therefore, having more than one option with varying designs and construction materials is necessary. The designs should have options for a twin pit on the one hand and a septic tank on the other hand. It is recommended that there may be an option for the larger pit size to dissuade the fear of it getting filled quickly. Moreover, there should be multiple options for superstructure: narrow, medium, and large.

A bathroom facility and water supply may be provided along with toilets. Otherwise, the households would not use toilets due to lack of water and use the toilets as the bathroom, which is a higher priority. Hence, there may also be an option for a toilet plus bathroom, including a water supply. Water supply should be included irrespective of demand for a bathroom facility. The government programme may also consider constructing more than one toilet for larger households. A single toilet in an enormous household excludes male members who continue open defecation. Having more than one toilet is also advisable if there is a higher percentage of female members in a household. It is common in villages for more than one family to reside in a single household or within the same premises. In such households, the number of toilets should equal the number of families residing in the household.

The implementation mechanism may be more efficient in places where payment delays are reported. The direct transfer of the reimbursement amount to beneficiaries' bank accounts is advisable, and government may construct toilets for weaker sections, old age, challenged, and dependent sections free of cost. The villagers may be more aware of the key persons, such as Swacchhatagrahi, for better contact and quick processing of applications. Recruitment and appointment of Swacchhatagrahi could be an important step in this direction, which would boost programme implementation and monitoring at the micro level.

Health and social workers should be more activated to motivate households for toilet construction and use. In many cases, toilets constructed under government programmes are not used for defecation for various reasons like shortage of water, uneasiness in using toilets, drainage problems, repair issues, etc. The health and social workers should play a pivotal role in ensuring that the households use the toilet. Households should be motivated and monitored even after the construction of toilets. Along with *swacchhagrahis*, other health and social workers may be incentivised to conduct these activities. Health workers' dissemination of general health information can make households aspire to better health. Prevention of waterborne diseases like cholera, typhoid, amoebiasis, diarrhoea, hepatitis, anaemia, urinary tract infections, and hookworm disease in children is possible only when villagers stop defecating in the open.

Change in sanitation behaviour is a collective activity. According to the WHO report (1 July 2021), 15% of the population of India is defecating in the open, comprising 1% of the urban population and 22% of the rural population. It is essential to appreciate the fact that the whole community has to stop defecating in the open; even if only a few persons defecate in the open, it will be almost impossible to stop the adverse effect of open defecation. Secondly, a continuation of open defecation by a few community members may trigger others to start defecting in the open. It may be helpful to develop informal norms for behavioural change. Joint monitoring by the community against open defecation could be a way forward to tackle the problem of open defecation. Fines may be imposed if someone is found defecating in the open. Public shaming by announcing the household details and local news channels, conditional sanctioning of Public Distribution System (PDS) are sanctioning strategies for dealing with open defecation. One the other hand, positive reinforcements such as providing water connections, and other basic services could also be one way to deal with the problem.

As using the toilet is an aspiration that develops with increasing living standards, the general cleanliness of households and locality may impact demand for sanitation positively. The villagers, especially the youth, may devote a specific amount of time daily for general cleanliness by participating in various voluntary activities, such as Swachh Bharat Summer Internship, Swachh Bharat Pakhwada, NSS, NCC, etc. The villages should have facilities like collection and disposal of waste and drainage facilities. It is advisable to form groups to conduct and monitor these activities. These collective efforts would, in turn, ensure bringing open defecation to an end.

Political Will. During the past 70 years, the sanitation interventions in India have not reached the expected outcomes. After initiating the Swachh Bharat Mission in 2014, the sanitation concept became a patriotism-linked national movement with the involvement of government departments. The political will to implement 100% defecation-free India was also an act of raising the public aspiration of making the nation a clean India. Political will be percolated down to the lowest level of officials, and public functionaries are one of the crucial determinants of sanitation coverage. However, the politicians may not make interventions at the household level. Politicians contacting the potential beneficiaries may put them under pressure and may distort the process of demand generation for sanitation. Health and social workers may be entrusted with motivating people to construct and use toilets. However, politicians may put more effort into monitoring the activities of these workers, such as adding sanitation as a mandate discussion agenda point in every Gram Sabha and SHG meeting. They may put more effort into IEC activities, organising drawing, singing, and elocution competitions in education institutions and involving NSS/NCC camps in targeted villages. Construction material should be made available more quickly. The government may find ways to implement the programme with cheaper local materials at a lower cost. The district-level public health engineering departments may be entrusted with research and development using cheaper local materials for construction and establishing manufacturing units in favour of SHG. Furthermore, cheaper chemicals for cleaning the toilets should be made available as the standard materials available in the market are costly, which would partially resolve the problems of foul smell and untidiness of toilets.

Sanitation as a Collective Activity

Change in sanitation behaviour is a collective activity. Individual household members, RI members, ASHA, AWW, and volunteers have a vital role in changing sanitation behaviour. Sanitation behaviour includes cleanliness, food hygiene, handwashing, ODF, and sewerage system. The community awareness of sanitation behaviour is low. People who have been forced to live in places with open sewage systems and engage in open defecation for generations have become accustomed to it, and it takes time to adjust to a new system. In India, approximately 62000 million litres of sewage are generated every day. Every day, 38722 million litres of untreated sewage are released, polluting water bodies and soil (Singh et al., 2020). Hence, the community should be accountable through formal and informal institutional mechanisms.

Moreover, it is also part of improving living standards and aspirational household goals. Hence, along with better income, households should be able to have better basic amenities. A safer and more convenient drinking water supply source is significant. It improves health standards and saves time for other value-added activities. Similarly, a well-built house improves living standards and is thus essential to changing sanitation behaviour (Panda & Padhi, 2017). Even a *pucca* road connecting the house or locality may positively impact the use of toilets. Hence, it is essential to make efforts to improve other basic services. A sanitation programme alone is unlikely to change sanitation behaviour.

Health and Sanitation Policies in India

Some consider the right to health as a necessary right for human beings. The right to health establishes a relationship between the right to life and living a dignified life that is non-discriminatory (Leary, 1994). It has been debatable whether the right to health is guaranteed under the fundamental rights, as it lacks enforceability and has been subject to interpretation by the higher judiciary. Many often contend that under Articles 14, 15, and 21 of the Constitution of India, which guarantees the right to life, equality and non-discrimination, health, drinking water, and reasonably good living conditions are guaranteed. Despite it being the subject of interpretation, successive governments in India have tried to enact laws and provisions to provide a dignified living for all its citizens. The challenges for universal healthcare for a country of India's proportion and the extreme poverty (Ravallion, 2008) are enormous. However, poor sanitation directly impacts the prevalence of diseases like diarrhoea, dengue, malaria, typhoid and hepatitis B and impacts per capita income and child mortality rate. Hence the Government of India initiated the National Health Policy in 1983, which promised health for all by 2000. However, in 2002, Government of India came up with a revised National Health Policy, which has been critiqued heavily because of its silence on the issues of comprehensive and universal primary health, which was part of the Alma-Ata Declaration (present-day Almaty in Kazakhstan) of 1978 (Gupta, 2002).

National Nutrition Policy (NNP). The inadequate access to potable water leads to less intake of nutrients and results in malnutrition in women and children. Half of the malnutrition cases in children are caused by improper sanitation and poor access to safe drinking water. In this concern, the Government of India has issued the National Nutrition Policy (NNP)[7] in 1993. The NNP policy deals with malnutrition issues among children, adolescent girls, pregnant and lactating mothers, and older adults. It emphasised various components like behaviour change, food fortification, low-cost nutrition food, food security, kitchen gardening, research, food adulteration, etc. To address the malnutrition issues among children under six years of age and lactating and pregnant women, the Poshan Abhiyan Scheme was introduced in 2017. It was intended to cover about 100 million beneficiaries by 2020.

Immunisation Program. Sanitation impacts on the immunity system to combat various diseases in children. In this context, the government focuses on sanitation infrastructure and immunisation. In this background, the government initiated the Expanded Program of Immunization (EPI) in 1978 to provide free vaccination, viz. diphtheria, polio, measles, tetanus, tuberculosis, hepatitis B, meningitis, and Pneumonia, among children.

Mission Indradhanush. Access to potable water, cleanliness, and sanitation will reduce the spread of infectious diseases and sustain natural immunity. In line with achieving complete immunisation coverage for mother and child, the Mission Indradhanush scheme was introduced in December 2014. The scheme has been implemented in four phases up to August 2017 and vaccinated about 68 lakh pregnant women and 2.5 crores of children. The scheme continues by revising the targets: Intensified Mission Indradhanush (IMM) and Intensified Mission Indradhanush 2.0 (IMM 2.0) and 3.0.

National Health Mission (NHM). Public health depends on the quality of sanitation, reducing the vulnerability to various diseases. In this context, to reinforce healthcare and sanitation for the people, the Government of India established the National Health Mission (NHM) in 2005. For effective implementation, the National Health Mission is decentralised into the National Rural Health Mission (NRHM) and the National Urban Health Mission (NUHM). This NHM is aimed to provide quality health services for reproductive, maternal, neo-natal, child, and adolescent health and communicable and non-communicable diseases. The NHM framework also focused a concurrent action on the improper sanitation root cause of many health problems.

Prevention of HIV/AIDS Act 2017. People living with HIV (PLHIV) are prone to diarrhoea and opportunistic diseases due to non-access to sanitation facilities, potable water, and hygienic food. It impacts the mortality rate of PLHIV. In 2019 there were 58.96 thousand PLHIV deaths in India. The Prevention of HIV/AIDS Act 2017 was enacted in April 2017 to improve the quality of life of PLHIV. The act emphasises protecting human rights, including avoiding stigma and discrimination, providing necessary care, support, and rehabilitation, strengthening grievances, and treating persons infected or affected with HIV/AIDS and healthcare providers. The Prevention of HIV/AIDS Act 2017 has also focused on eliminating discrimination in accessing proper sanitation facilities, including community water resources and toilets.

Health Insurance. In line with safeguarding public health and sanitation, the government has been introducing various health insurance schemes to exclude medical expenditures and provide quality treatment facilities to ordinary people. About 17 government health insurance schemes are existent in India.

Policies on Sanitation. Since its independence, the Government of India has progressively been giving priority to sanitation by considerable investing in sanitation infrastructure and enacting various laws, policies, and schemes by involving the state and local government to achieve sustainable sanitation. The following significant schemes have been implemented on a large scale after independence.

The Prohibition of Employment as Manual Scavengers and Their Rehabilitation (Act and Rule). The immoral practice of engaging manual scavengers and constructing or using dry toilets in the twenty-first century is a blemish on the nation's status. The manual scavengers engage in cleaning dry toilets, sewers, and railway stations. While they were engaging in this inhuman job, about 1760 deaths of manual scavengers happened across the nation. The scavengers engaging in sewers and toilet cleaning come in direct contact with human excreta, which they physically remove. It is a highly shameful and cruel practice that has been perpetuated in the country for generations. They are most prone to accidental deaths while involved in cleaning work. Also, they are vulnerable to lung-related diseases like TB, asthma, bronchitis, and nausea. In 1993, the Government of India passed an act prohibiting employment as manual scavengers and their rehabilitation to secure the health and dignity of scavengers.

Total Sanitation Campaign (TSC)

To access the sanitation programmes for all districts in the nation, the Government of India has intervened Total Sanitation Campaign (TSC) in 1999 as one of the world's most extensive rural sanitation programmes. The scheme generated demand for sanitary facilities by introducing financial incentives for constructing toilets, developing information, education, and communication (IEC) materials, and disseminating knowledge and capacity-building strategies.

School Sanitation and Hygiene Education (SSHE) Programme. The poor sanitation facilities in schools would induce various diseases among schoolgoing children and impact dropouts. Therefore the schools' usage of toilets is significant for promoting sanitation behaviour among children. This programme was started in 1999 and implemented under the Total Sanitation Campaign (TSC). A key objective of this programme is to facilitate toilet construction in every school and inculcate handwashing and hygiene education for schoolchildren.

Nirmal Gram Puraskar (NGP). Most of the sanitation activities introduced by the government have been visible in urban areas, and significant blocks, but the village-level sanitation has become challenging since the inception of sanitation interventions made by the government. In this outlook, to offer complete sanitation services to far-flung villages, the Government of India introduced the Nirmal Gram Puraskar (NGP) scheme in October 2003 across the nation. Every year the Nirmal Gram Puraskar (NGP) was awarded to selected villages, including cash prizes ranging from Rs 50000 to Rs 500000. The selection parameters for beneficiary villages are individual household toilets, sanitation in schools, and Anganwadis, access to potable water, IEC, and solid and liquid waste management. Research suggests that Nirmal Gram Puraskar has been a trigger for developing a competitive spirit in sanitation among the Grama Panchayats (GPs). Because of the incentive, the GP leadership has taken a personal interest in focusing on increasing the coverage of households and schools in rural areas (George, 2009).

National Urban Sanitation Policy (NUSP). To strengthen the sanitation activities at the urban level, the Ministry of Urban Development started the National Urban Sanitation Policy (NUSP) in 2008. This policy is aimed to promote comprehensive sanitation strategies such as capacity building for urban local bodies, sanitation behaviour, ODF cities, waste management, and innovations.

National Rural Drinking Water Program (NRDWP). Access to safe drinking water is a primary right of every citizen. Many rural areas were under water crisis and frequently faced various waterborne diseases. As a result, child mortality rates also surged. Following this significant public health issue, in 2009, the Government of India launched the National Rural Drinking Water Program (NRDWP). The reasoning was that safe drinking water would prevent different waterborne diseases. Thus, the objective was to provide a safe and adequate amount of drinking water for every household in rural areas. The National Rural Drinking Water Program (NRDWP) had formulated a piped drinking water supply policy to encourage the ODF villages.

Solid Waste Management Rules, 2016. Solid waste management is part of providing comprehensive sanitation dealing with waste material generated daily. Every day, 0.15 million metric tonnes (MT) of domestic and non-domestic wastage are collected in India. The processing and dumping have become a challenge as 15000 metric tonnes of garbage are disposed of daily, and 5.5 million tonnes of solid waste are disposed of in open areas yearly. About 20% of solid waste is processed, and 80% of solid waste is dumped in open or landfills. Solid and plastic waste disposal significantly affects air and land pollution. Apart from notifying the dumping area, rehabilitation after dumping needs to follow eco-friendly guidelines. The waste materials need to be processed, segregated, recycled, and dumped by technical procedures to reduce the environmental pollution hazards. Without following the appropriate procedures for dumping solid waste, air pollution, water pollution, soil pollution, and resource exploitation would occur. So there is a need to frame uniform guidelines, rules, and laws to protect the global environment. In India, the Solid Waste Management (SWM) Rules were framed in 2016 for directing criteria for establishing solid waste processing units, geographical specifications areas, waste energy process, sanitary landfills, measurements, closure and rehabilitation, selection of dumping yards, buffer zones, facilities creation in sanitary landfills, etc.

Faecal Sludge and Septage Management (FSSM). The Government of India formulated the national policy on Faecal Sludge and Septage Management (FSSM) in 2017. The policy directives to set up the treatment plants and streamline the sewage system in coordination with local bodies exist all over India's urban areas. As part of the comprehensive sanitation process, the collection, emptying, transportation, disposal, treatment, and reuse of the faecal sludge from individual households and public toilets is a challenging task for the nation to prevent contamination of water bodies and soil and air pollution. With the limited workforce and infrastructure for disposing of the faecal matter, about 70% of the human excreta has been dumped in the open places, leading to severe contamination of water bodies and agriculture fields and causing health hazards for human beings. Hence to streamline the imbalance and adverse effects, the Bill and Melinda foundation facilitated the alliance for National Faecal Sludge and Septage Management (NFSSM) in 2016. This alliance is aimed to support the activities meant for sanitation at different levels. The alliance collaborated with ministries like the Ministry of Housing and Urban Affairs (MoHUA) and the Department of Drinking Water and Sanitation (DWS) and worked to evolve a national policy on FSSM in 2017.

Policies on Water Management. In May 2019, the Government of India merged the Department of Drinking Water and Sanitation and Department of Water Resources, River Development and Ganga Rejuvenation under the Ministry of Jal Shakthi. This mission also monitors sanitation through waste management in rural India. To provide potable water for all households' drinking and domestic needs in the rural area, the Ministry of Jal Shakthi is operating the National Rural Drinking Water Program (NRDWP) and the Jal Jeevan Mission. As part of comprehensive sanitation, the National Rural Drinking Water Program (NRDWP) was initiated in 2009 to offer sufficient water for drinking, cooking, and other domestic needs, i.e., 55 litres per capita per day. The programme aims to reduce waterborne diseases and reduce child mortality and public health burden significantly.

Jal Jeevan Mission. The unsafe drinking water leads to many waterborne infections and affects public health and mortality rate. In these circumstances, the Government of India has restructured the National Rural Drinking Water Program (NRDWP) into the Jal Jeevan Mission, aimed to provide potable drinking water for every rural household and public institution in a sustainable approach by 2024. The Jal Jeevan Mission supports the local government in establishing adequate water supply to every rural household through Functional Household Tap connection (FHTC). The Jal Jeevan Mission also focuses on sanitation and greywater management as water is the primary resource for ODF interventions. Despite all constraints, due to the continuous policy interventions and proportionately larger budgetary support since independence, drinking water is available to more than 92% of the population (Cronin et al., 2016).

Atal Mission for Rejuvenation and Urban Transformation (AMRUT). As part of providing potable drinking water for urban communities, the Housing and Urban Affairs Ministry has implemented the Atal Mission for Rejuvenation and Urban Transformation (AMRUT) scheme since June 2015. The objective of this programme was to provide safe water with the aim of 139 lakh tap water connections. The AMRUT scheme is initiated with a Rs 77640 crores budget. It includes allied water management activities, i.e., management of water bodies, sewerages, rejuvenation of existing water systems, water treatment plants, groundwater and overhead tanks, etc.

Literature Gap

The above review informs us of the sanitation programmes launched in the country, both success and failure stories. One common theme in the literature is having substantial sociocultural factors on the community, both detrimental and driving forces of sanitation. It also informs us that the interventions increased the usage and awareness of sanitation in society. Though the main objective of sanitation through information, education, and communication (IEC) is to raise people's awareness, it may result in demand. However, people demanding the toilet as an outcome of awareness and behaviour changes have limited space. However, demand in this context differs from supply and demand's economic terms. Demand is a determinant of change through the construction of toilets as part of the sanitation campaign. It can be noted that the number of toilets has increased – as part of the sanitation programmes – without demand made by the target population or villagers.

It should be noted that when the programme became target-oriented in terms of the number of toilets constructed, the officials focused on the construction of toilets while ignoring the fundamental requirement of focussing on information, education, and communication strategies and mobilising people for collective action against open defecation. Motivational measures were largely ignored. The various research studies' findings focus on the subsidy and construction, whereas behaviour changes and determinants on the part of the community and individuals have been largely overlooked. The guidelines of the Total Sanitation Campaign (TSC) and Nirmal Bharat Abhiyan (NBA) mention interpersonal communication for behaviour change, but it is rarely executed. Most of these reports and studies also mentioned the deficiencies in implementation but rarely explored the challenges and problems facing sanitation promotion.

Given the significance of diversity in Indian society, understanding the local context and challenges arising out of it becomes critical for any meaningful intervention both at the policy and implementation stage. Every village in India poses some unique challenges and opportunities in terms of soil conditions, availability of material, and emotional triggers for motivating people to change behaviour at the individual level and collective mobilisation. Thus, leveraging the unique knowledge of the community in terms of soil conditions, water drainage, materials availability, and construction methods is essential in developing a sustainable model. Ignorance of these factors is likely to lead to failures. In light of this, the primary research reflects on the local aspects of sanitation by locating the local cultural practices that can be detrimental and progressive. In its effort, the research explores the psychological aspects of the people towards sanitation.

3 Current Scenario and Regional Variations

Background to the Swachh Bharat Mission

With the Swachh Bharat Mission (SBM), the country witnessed a silent revolution in constructing toilets, covering an additional 10.52% of rural households, with more than 63000 villages being declared open defecation free (ODF). However, to understand the trajectory of SBM, one must delve deeper into the context from which SBM emerged.

Decentralisation of Water Supply and Sanitation[1]

The water supply and sanitation sector has been given enormous emphasis recently as part of the global programme on poverty alleviation. These services directly impact human development and indirectly impact economic growth. Decentralising the water supply and sanitation sector has provided sustainable community-managed infrastructure in Third-World nations. In many developing countries, decentralisation has already been initiated in the water supply and sanitation. India is no exception in this regard. This chapter will examine the water supply and sanitation schemes, the delivery structure, and the decentralisation experience in rural India. Additionally, we would review some international decentralisation experiences in water supply and sanitation delivery. We have also attempted to determine the factors leading to the success or failure of decentralisation in water supply and sanitation services.

Providing safe drinking water and sanitation in India's rural areas is the responsibility of the respective states. However, the central government supplements the effort of the state government to provide these services through Centrally Sponsored Schemes (CSS). States generally plan, design, and execute water supply schemes (and often continue to operate) through their State Public Health Engineering Department (or, as in the case of some states, Panchayati Raj Engineering Departments or Rural Development Engineering Departments) and Water Boards.

After the 73rd constitutional amendment, water supply and sanitation were included in the Eleventh Schedule of the Constitution.[2] States can entrust these functions to the Panchayats, which has opened the possibility of planning and delivering services in a demand-driven decentralised structure rather than a

DOI: 10.4324/9781032726267-3

supply-driven centralised structure as earlier. The major problem with the centralised implementation of water supply and sanitation schemes in India is that the planning process is supply-driven rather than demand-driven. The schemes, in recent years, have ignored user preferences and their ability to pay for different service levels. The planning process overlooks the need for maintenance, rehabilitation, and rejuvenation of existing facilities. The block-level executive engineer assesses water requirements and other constraints at the ground and plans for water supply at the end-user level. The assessment is then translated into a proposal for a new and augmented scheme and passed to the executive or superintending engineer for administrative approval. Here, what is warranted is a demand-oriented and client-responsive approach where communities will have access to relevant information and will exercise control or oversight at each stage of planning and implementation (World Bank, 1998a). User financing and cost recovery are also needed for additional coverage and quality improvements. The budget is only enough to meet expenses for replacing old systems, operations, and maintenance (Pushpangadan & Murugan, 1998).

The institutional structure of water supply and sanitation services delivery has also been centralised in other developing countries during the 1980s. Centrally managed water supply and sanitation programmes used to be conventional engineering solutions. It resulted in infrastructure beyond the people's capacity to maintain. When the governments faced hard budget constraints, water supplies fell into disrepair, and people could not repair them (WSP, 2003). In this backdrop, community-oriented management of water supply and sanitation has been encouraged in the 1990s in these countries. However, the experience of decentralisation is not identical in all the countries. On the other hand, there are also commonalities in the key factors determining the outcome.

Rural Sanitation Schemes in India

India's primary water supply and sanitation schemes originate with the central government, while state governments partially contribute. The delivery mechanism of services primarily depends on the state governments. However, in sanitation, it is mainly determined by the central government. One of the earlier programmes on sanitation (the Central Rural Sanitation Programme) was launched after realising that without a proper sanitation programme in rural areas, the intended benefits of the water supply programme in rural areas cannot be achieved. Therefore, the rural sanitation and water supply programmes were nurtured as twin programmes. The Central Rural Sanitation Programme (CRSP) was highly subsidised. It provided full subsidy for constructing sanitary toilets for scheduled castes, scheduled tribes, and landless workers. The programme had two significant lacunas; one, it gave full subsidy to specific sections of the village community but was not open to all communities. The problem with the approach is that open defecation will continue when all the residents are not covered. The chances of water contamination remain high, and all problems related to contaminated water continue.

Moreover, people who have already constructed toilets may not use them because of the prevailing social norm of open defecation (because a section is still without toilets at home). Two, the programme emphasised a single model of toilet, a twin pit, pour or flush system with brick masonry construction. The total cost was about Rs. 2500. However, the toilet design was impervious to the local climatic and soil conditions and the economic conditions of the target group, which resulted in a low level of adoption. Secondly, a programme that focused only on specific categories of rural population with opportunities to subsidise only a few toilets in villages opened up the scope for patronisation and unethical practices that affected the programme quality (Gunyon, 1998).

Given the inherent problems mainly due to the programme design and implementation issues, a new programme was launched in 1999 under 'Total Sanitation Campaign (TSC)'. The programme was envisaged to be people-centric. Unlike its predecessor programme, it aimed at people who came forward or volunteered to construct the toilet, which considered the local conditions like climate, soil, and household-level financial conditions to have a place-specific suitable toilet design. Some people referred it to a community-led model; however, it fell short of that as the subsidy amount was meant for the below poverty line (BPL) families in the village and not open to all villagers. Secondly, the subsidy was available for the low-cost model (Rs. 2200). In the case of excess cost over Rs. 2500 the household constructing the toilet was required to pay from their resources; the state governments were allowed to provide extra subsidy from the state government funds. One significant departure of the Total Sanitation Campaign (TSC) was its strong focus on Information, Education, and Communication (IEC) to generate demand from the target group to construct toilets.

The Total Sanitation Campaign (TSC) was a centrally sponsored scheme. The state government has to provide matching contributions under the Minimum Needs Programme (MNP). Financial support in a 20% subsidy is given to construct individual toilets for the BPL households. Schools were provided financial assistance to construct toilets. For co-educational schools, the construction of separate toilets for boys and girls was emphasised. It was the same for the Anganwadis and Balwadis. Wherever land was available, community sanitary complexes for women were proposed in villages, and the community became responsible for its management.

Delivery Structure of Sanitation in India

In India, rural water supply services have been decentralised in various states. The activity transferred to different levels of Panchayat for rural water supply also is different from one state to another. However, the delivery mechanism of sanitation is almost the same across states since the centre determines the mechanism. Given the differential in rural water supply delivery mechanisms across states, we have chosen only one state to examine the rural water supply and sanitation delivery mechanism. A state with a long history of decentralisation, mainly rural water supply and sanitation, would be most suitable for study. In this respect, West Bengal is the most appropriate state since rural water supply and sanitation were delegated to the Panchayats in 1973 (De, 2009). In various cases, the Panchayat Samitis (PSs) have been empowered to adopt different schemes, including financial assistance, for developing water supply and sanitation and related matters in the interest of public health. Similar power has also been given to the Zilla Parishad (ZP). In addition, ZP has been given the power to advise the state government on all matters relating to the development work in Gram Panchayats (GPs) and Panchayat Samitis under its jurisdiction.

Rural sanitation is one of the critical components of hygiene promotion and avoiding many deadly diseases. After restructuring the Central Rural Sanitation Programme (CRSP), the Total Sanitation Campaign (TSC) was launched in 1999 following a community-led and people-centred approach. It is a centrally sponsored scheme, and the state government provides the matching grant under MNP. For different activities of TSC, the ratio of matching grants is different. The centre provides the entire fund for start-up activities. It is a demand-driven programme involving non-government organisations (NGOs) and Gram Panchayat. Beneficiaries contribute to this programme; about 20% subsidy is provided only to the BPL population. In West Bengal, TSC was closely coordinated with UNICEF and Panchayat and Rural Development Department. UNICEF supported the State Sanitation Cell, helped in IEC activities, and gave technological assistance. At the district level, a standing committee on Public Health and Environment (Janaswasthya O Paribesh Sthayee Samiti) and District Sanitation Cell worked in close coordination in monitoring and evaluation, supervision of sanitary mart, etc. At the block level, a similar standing committee is there for monitoring and evaluation, quality control, etc. However, despite many structurally facilitative conditions, research evidence from the district of Birbhum in West Bengal suggests that there have been many pitfalls in extending the coverage of sanitation services progress in the state. One of the major drawbacks has been a meagre allocation of funds, and perhaps because of it, very low utilisation of funds has occurred. The demand from the users has been deficient, which may be partly attributed to the negligence of the Panchayat officials and the inactivity of ground-level motivators. Thus, there has been a low demand for sanitary materials. The cost of the toilet and the grant received from the government did not match. Most people could not generate the finance needed to construct a toilet at home. However, there was a lack of awareness about sanitation and the necessity of having toilets; this was also highlighted by the fact that there was lower participation by villagers in government-initiated meetings related to sanitation (De, 2010).

Rural Sanitary Marts

Additionally, Rural Sanitary Marts (RSMs) were set up to meet the demand for construction material for toilets across the country. RSMs were considered an integral part of the centrally sponsored TSC scheme. In 1991 the RSMs were launched by the Uttar Pradesh government with the active support of UNICEF. RSM outlets sold the construction materials and also helped people in designing toilets.

Rural Sanitary Mart (RSM) was the key institution in TSC. RSM is constructed after Panchayat Samiti (PS) approves it and sends its recommendation to the Zilla Parishad (ZP). ZP, in turn, approves it and sends the recommendation to the Panchayat and Rural Development Department. At first, ZP provides initial funds for constructing marts (marts are supposed to have their land). Then ZP provides a revolving fund for production. Later, the Block Development Office (BDO) apprises the progress of the work done (progress of marts) to ZP, and ZP releases funds accordingly. ZP also distributed funds for IEC, which was routed through the Block Development Office (BDO); the eligible households could claim the subsidy amount from the Block Development Office (BDO).

Rural Sanitary Mart (RSM) worked closely with a Non-Government Organisation (NGO) and Panchayati Raj institutions. The Gram Panchayat (GP) was primarily responsible for contacting the RSM and monitoring work progress. RSM consisted of two mart managers, two motivators, and two masons. For every 150–200 households, one motivator motivated people to construct a toilet. Additionally, the motivator prepared the list of households participating in the programme and collected their contributions. They got a commission for the construction of each toilet. The RSMs also set the target and make a production plan. They were responsible for the supply of materials, the construction of toilets, and campaigning and demand generation for hygiene promotion in collaboration with the Panchayats and the non-government organisations (NGOs). It is done through wall writing, leaflet, folksong, VDO show, magic, puppet show, household visits, group meeting, cinema slide, play, etc. Overall, RSM takes care of the demand and supply side of constructing toilets. The details of the structure of functioning RSM are given in Figure 3.1.

Sanitation Sector in West Bengal

The distribution mechanism at the district and block levels is unclear. IEC activity has not been given enough importance, as evident from the state government's ad hoc and sporadic implementation of the IEC. Without proper IEC, problems of supply-driven programmes may get transmitted to the demand-driven programmes partially due to the IEC's role in capacity building at the grassroots-level workers involved in implementing the programme. Moreover, the simultaneous existence of both supply-driven and demand-driven programmes may create confusion and make the delivery system less transparent.

Panchayat Samiti and Gram Panchayat have an enormous responsibility in TSC. The programmes are demand-driven, where the Panchayati Raj Institutions (PRIs) create demand for the services by building hygiene consciousness. PRIs may not give enough effort to building consciousness since it is politically less attractive as benefits may not be immediately tangible. If the PRIs try to implement these programmes without building the consciousness, the objective of creating a demand-driven programme will be defeated. The problem of a supply-driven system will get transferred to the demand-driven system. Interviews with beneficiaries during May–July 2005 in Birbhum district of West Bengal revealed that awareness

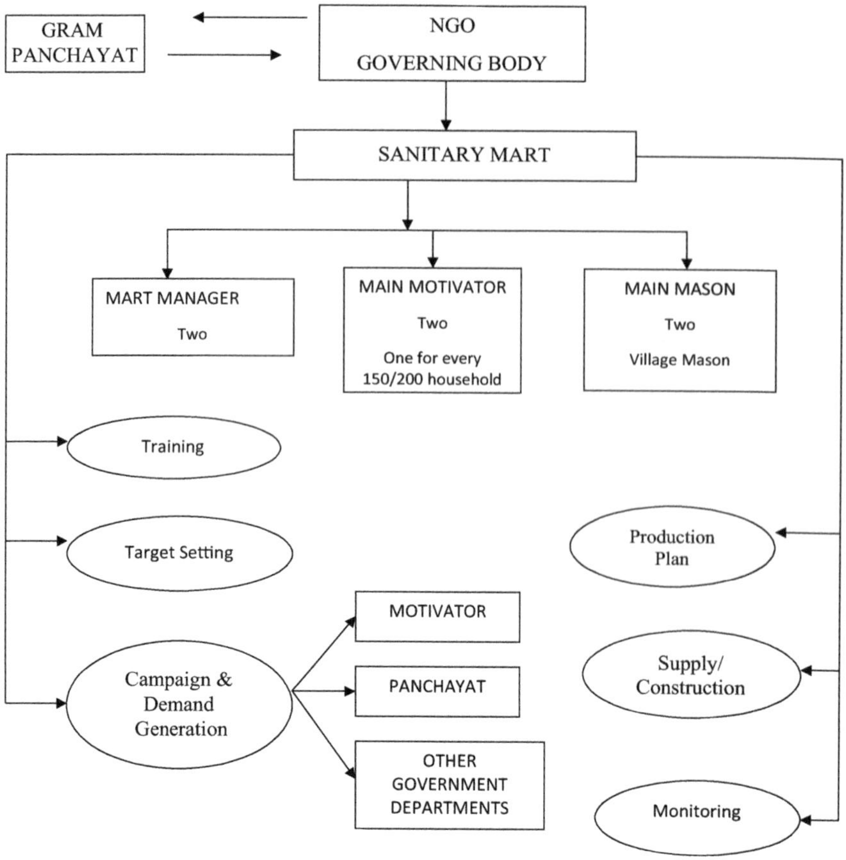

Figure 3.1 Structure of Functioning of Sanitary Mart.

Source: Panchayat and Rural Development Department, West Bengal

generated for TSC, particularly in Swajaldhara, is weak. Beneficiaries are, in many cases, obliged to contribute to sanitation rather than creating demand on their own.

Moreover, the toilets provided were of substandard quality, and people were unwilling to use them. These became sunk investments by the government and the households. Evaluation regarding satisfaction and preference of people has not been done till now. In TSC, institutional weakness arose mainly because of a lack of effort in demand generation. Difficulty in the disbursement of the subsidy from the BDO and the non-profitability of marts also weakened the scheme's progress.

Decentralisation in the Water Supply and Sanitation: Indian Experience

Decentralisation in India's water supply and sanitation sector has suffered from low community participation, low capacity at the local level, weak coordination between different government departments, and elite capture. The water resource sector review of the World Bank (1998a) has identified several problems in the decentralisation process in the sector. First, the split in the responsibility between administrative levels has resulted in poor performance. Second, the weak coordination between public health and Zilla Parishad engineering departments and delays in financial and technical approvals and sanctions impede implementation. The third problem is the weak interaction of state and district agencies with the Panchayats limiting the higher administrative levels to recover dues from the Panchayats. These problems arise because of the wide distribution of responsibilities across agencies and unclear lines of accountability. Other problems are poor hydrological investigations, a relatively higher percentage of improper design, cost overruns, and limited quality assurance despite a comprehensive set of built-in controls. Thus, the weakness of the supply-driven approach is transferred to the districts and local agencies.

Studies have strengthened the suspicion on the functioning of Panchayats on the ground that decentralisation has strengthened the vested interests in the rural areas. The socio-economic strength of the Panchayat leaders has played a significant role in this regard. The establishment of user groups (i.e. Village Water Supply and Sanitation Committees) with the legal backing of Panchayats may solve these problems, as has occurred in Karnataka (World Bank, 1998b). A proper demand-driven approach with coordination between the Panchayats and Village Water Supply and Sanitation Committees will provide services that the households will be willing to pay for. The NGOs or private sector agencies may also provide some technical support.

Moreover, suspicion on the functioning has been raised that the Gram Panchayats have little autonomy to implement their programmes. The central and state governments continue to control the day-to-day functioning of the Panchayats in the guise of legislative control over grants. The main problem of the local governments is the lack of financial resources. Gram Panchayats are entitled to levy and collect taxes, but the collection rate is typically low for water charges and other government levies. The other major problem the decentralisation process faces is a lack of capacity.

Comparing the efficiency of water utilities under the control of the state and the local government in terms of expenses and asset utilisation in Madhya Pradesh and Chhattisgarh, Asthana (2003) has found that efficiency is higher in centralised utilities than in decentralised utilities. The efficiency measures considered are the mean of operating expenses scaled by annual production and production of potable water divided by assets. The author argued that the engineering and technical skills required are less readily available at the district and gram panchayat levels than the state-level implementation under the decentralised management. Secondly, funds flow from the state government to the districts, and the gram panchayat level, is not on time and is very meagre. Most importantly, there is rampant corruption at the local level, and massive leakage of funds occurs – this is done in cahoots with the local elites.

Various evidence suggests that efficiency in rural sanitation increases when the participation of beneficiaries increases in construction and maintenance. In

Karnataka Integrated Rural Water Supply and Environmental Sanitation Schemes, community participation has played a significant role in planning, implementation, operation, and maintenance (Veerashekharappa, 2000). The community has borne 30% of the capital costs of environmental sanitation. It has mobilised resources to operate and maintain assets by collecting connection fees and water tariffs fixed by a locally developed institution – the Village Water Supply Committee (VWSC). Consultants were appointed to promote community participation and impart skills to the community during the planning and implementation stage before operation and maintenance were transferred to VWSCs. For fixing the water tariff, the cross-subsidy mechanism was adopted. The efficient functioning of the project in terms of the quality and timely construction of the water supply schemes is directly proportional to the strength of community participation. The evidence suggested that if people's sense of ownership is reduced, their commitment to maintaining the assets and the ability of the VWSCs to function sustainably would be eroded. So generating a sense of equal ownership will likely contribute to the programme's efficiency. It is possible through equal participation in the decision-making by every community member. On the other hand, efficiency in service delivery itself has ensured greater participation.

A study on the Second Maharashtra Rural Water Supply Sanitation Project in the tribal areas of Maharashtra elicits some important observations (GOM, 1998). It has been observed that the Village Panchayat's functioning usually is greatly influenced by a few rich and powerful people who shape the agenda by keeping their interests in mind. As a result, the communities neither participate nor are consulted. Activities of the Panchayats are generally concentrated only in main villages rendering the hamlets neglected. Panchayats are also urged to select costly options to benefit from a higher share. Tribal men and women strongly desire that all decisions related to technological options, delivery design, household contributions, operation and maintenance, etc. are made and executed at the hamlet level rather than at the Village Panchayat level. Though the central concern for tribal men is affordability, they are also concerned about participation, transparency, accountability, and much-needed capacity building.

Other evidence also suggests that community participation is key to success in decentralisation in this sector. The World Bank Impact Evaluation Study in Karnataka, Maharashtra, and Rajasthan suggested an absence of meaningful community participation, which results from unclear roles and responsibilities of village communities and committees, NGOs, and local governments. Further, there was no clear line of demarcation of roles and responsibilities of these institutions, which resulted in lower cost recovery (World Bank, 1998b). As a result, the project-provided opportunity for community development was wasted, and sustained operation of the system is unlikely and uncertain. In the case of Karnataka, although the social capital indicators are better, the influence of Zilla Panchayat in charge of implementation and political interference by local government have undermined the effort of community participation. As a result, cost recovery indicators are low. Cost recovery is crucial as it imparts a sense of ownership of assets within the community. In Rajasthan, recovery of the organisation and management cost of the project was not realised due to the lack of actual ownership of the ultimate beneficiaries. They neither had control over any resources nor were influenced in decision-making.

On the other hand, project performance is highly satisfactory in the Swajal Project, where the community, with the help of NGOs, has made informed choices about technology and level of service (Iyer, 1998). Since the cost is a significant factor in decision-making, choosing the technology after a feasibility study is vital to cover capital costs and accept the full responsibility for operation and maintenance costs. The community, in this case, has controlled construction funds through a joint account with an NGO. Transparency in the system has been restored through NGOs by providing information to the community and explaining the game's rules. NGOs helped to strengthen community capacity. A powerful sense of village ownership has been observed as the Village Water and Sanitation Committee (VWSC) has owned the facilities created.

The above case studies suggest that community participation in water supply and sanitation projects is most important in achieving efficiency of service delivery and equity in the distribution of benefits. In turn, community participation will increase when the service is efficient and satisfies the expectation of all sections of beneficiaries. Moreover, participation will increase only when the community gets a sense of ownership and dignity. Cost sharing in terms of money or labour could impart this sense. In the initial phase, building capacity and generating consciousness are most important for participation. NGOs can become instrumental in helping them in this respect.

Decentralisation of Sanitation Management: International Experience

This section discusses experiences from a few developing countries on decentralisation in water supply and sanitation. The countries chosen are Ghana, South Africa, Lesotho, Malawi, Uganda, Zimbabwe, and Ethiopia. Water supply and sanitation decentralisation in these countries started mainly in the 1990s.

In Ghana, Community Water and Sanitation Agency (CWSA) was created in 1998 and acted as a coordinator and facilitator of community-managed water supplies rather than an implementer (WSP, 2003). In South Africa, a community water supply and sanitation policy was adopted in 1994 (WSP, 2003), which provided the foundation for the legislative and regulatory framework of the Water Services Act 1997. As a result, water supply and sanitation coverage increased from below to above sub-Saharan Africa's average after 2000. Though sanitation is lagging, water supply coverage has progressed a lot. The sanitation programme in Lesotho was initiated in the early 1980s (WSP, 2003). Institutional arrangements at the national and district levels involved communities in the planning and managing of sanitation programmes. The government prioritised its effort on education and promotion. Rural sanitation coverage increased from a mere 15% in the 1980s to more than 50% in 2000.

Malawi is going through a decentralisation process to devolve administration and political authority from the central ministries to districts. But the decentralisation process is still relatively new (Slaymaker & Newborne, 2004). District staff generally feel more accountable to the central ministry than District Assemblies, whose resources undermine authority. Each district has a District Development Fund (DDF) and prepares a three-year District Development Plan, a central key element of decentralisation in Malawi. It has been found that the link of District Development Plans downwards to individual village-level and upwards to national-level planning process has remained weak. Moreover, District Assemblies lack the capacity and authority to coordinate and regulate sectoral investment. DDF and District Assemblies are not involved in selecting, implementing, or monitoring investments.

The process of decentralising the water supply and sanitation sector was started in 1995 in Uganda by establishing community-managed water and sanitation services through Water User Committees and Associations (Slaymaker & Newborne, 2004). Further elaborating on the principles of the demand-driven approach, a new water policy consistent with the decentralisation policy was finalised in 1999. After these initiatives, it has been observed that decentralisation has increased inequity. There are four levels of rural local government in Uganda. They are District, Sub-counties, Parishes, and Villages. Inequity in the distribution of water points has been observed at the level of Sub-county and Parish. The inequity in distribution between Sub-countries and Parishes has also increased. It has been found that the relative inequity in the distribution of water points is universally greater between lower levels of local governments, Parish, than between upper levels of local government, Sub-county.

Decentralisation in Zimbabwe was initiated to redress colonial disparities between large-scale commercial farming areas and communal areas by fostering the participation of local people in development activities beneficial to them (Makumbe, 1996). It has been observed that decentralisation efforts were unsuccessful due to wide-scale poverty and lack of capacity (Mtisi & Nicol, 2003). In Ethiopia, water and sanitation infrastructure is provided primarily by local government (Woredas) and the non-government sector, with central and regional governments accounting for under 4% of total water supply and sanitation expenditure (WSP, 2003). The decentralisation efforts did not yield any positive outcome due to a lack of capacity building at the ground level.

The above discussion reveals that the decentralisation experience in developing countries is mixed. In Ghana, South Africa, and Lesotho, water supply and sanitation decentralisation has increased coverage. However, decentralisation has led to declining water supply services deliveries in other countries like Malawi, Uganda, Zimbabwe, and Ethiopia. Factors that have been identified to be most important in determining the impact of decentralisation are political accountability, people's participation, transparency, policy coherence, and capacity at the lower level. We have discussed all these factors separately.

Political Accountability and People's Participation

Political commitment has been the major factor behind this success of decentralisation in Ghana. The national mood of change in the country's political economy in the 1980s favoured reform and innovation in water supply and sanitation. Successive governments of different parties have seen water and sanitation as essential contributors to social and economic development. Legislation has also clearly defined most policies and roles of different agencies within the sector. In South Africa, the critical factor behind the successful implementation of decentralised water supply and sanitation programmes is the commitment of political leaders. The Department of Water Affairs and Forestry (DWAF), the government department in charge of water supply and sanitation, has changed its function from implementation to support and regulation. Local political leaders have also played a vital role. They have been involved in setting budget priorities, service delivery standards, and approving projects. Legislation has also played an essential role by encompassing extensive social and economic rights, including essential water and sanitation.

The sanitation programme of Lesotho is yet another example of a successful decentralisation experience due to high political accountability. Though the original impetus for the sanitation programme came from sector professionals and external agencies, politicians also played an essential role by recognising the sanitation programme's importance and allocating significant sums to sanitation through the government's regular budget. The district sanitation teams have been entrusted with the central role of implementation. In the case of Lesotho, the evolving legal framework gave legitimacy to the sanitation programme's position as a regular part of the public sector's work. Communities have also managed sanitation services through technical and professional support from private sector companies. Media also helped in generating people's demand for sanitation.

Transparency and Policy Coherence

In Malawi, poor coordination and planning have led to inequities in resource allocation, with investment significantly greater in already well-served areas than poorly served areas. It has also led to water points becoming not functional due to a lack of maintenance by the community. The fragmented nature of water sector developments has led to a lack of policy coherence, which has led to poor coordination between different actors in sectoral investment, adoption of inappropriate technology, and confusion among beneficiary populations regarding the role and responsibilities of different institutions.

In Uganda, due to a poorly coordinated planning process and inadequate performance measures and tools, district and sub-countries' local planning and budgetary decisions are highly iniquitous and unsustainable. The division of roles between community, sub-county, and district for operation and maintenance is unclear, and no fund is allocated. The decentralisation process in Ghana is slower – because the local government organisations lack the requisite expertise in discharging their new role. The Community Water and Sanitation Agency (CWSA) has been formed to implement water programmes on behalf of many local governments as a temporary measure. At the same time, it has been given the charge of helping and supporting local government to take on implementation work. The small private sector, NGOs, and media have been supporting them. However, CWSA and politicians were unwilling to accept the help offered by the small private sector, NGOs, and media.

Local governments' financial and operational capacity has also been observed in South Africa, with a significant proportion of local governments not ready to take on their legal obligation for water and sanitation. Communities have been given technical and professional support to manage sanitation. Civil society organisations and media have also played an essential role in public scrutiny and transparency of water programmes. In Ethiopia, the local government, Woredas, is also constrained by capacity due to the lack of trained personnel. Lack of money and lack of access to spare parts or technical skills are significant constraints in Malawi's decentralisation. Lack of access to credit or banking facilities aggravates this problem.

In Uganda, it has also been found that the socio-economic status of a sub-county is probably a significant factor in both its ability to attract new investment in water and sanitation and its capacity to operate and maintain the facilities once established. In Zimbabwe, it has been observed that communities cannot contribute monthly water fees due to poverty. Moreover, they withheld their financial contribution to the water point committee because of concerns over funds management. In many areas, people do not know about village and ward assemblies. The participation of external institutions like NGOs often aggravates local-level complexities and defeats the premise of community management of water sources.

In India, the major stumbling block in the progress of decentralisation is the existing centralised structure of delivery of services. In the case of sanitation, though the programme is demand-driven, the government also sets specific targets, which are entrusted to the local government, which propels the local governments to take the seat of implementer rather than being a promoter of sanitation facilities. The experience of decentralisation in India shows that community participation is the primary factor behind the success of the sanitation sector. Apart from this, weak coordination between government departments, including Panchayats and village water supply committees, makes the line of accountability ambiguous and thus discourages community participation.

Decentralisation experience of rural water supply and sanitation in less developed countries reveals that political accountability, people's participation, transparency, policy coherence, capacity at the lower level, and monitoring and evaluation are the main factors behind these programmes. In Ghana, South Africa, and Lesotho, political accountability is the key to success. In Malawi, Uganda, and Ethiopia, lack of policy coherence and transparency is the most critical factor behind the low performance of the schemes. The lack of financial and operational capacity at the lower level in many countries studied above has also hindered the progress of the schemes delivered in a decentralised institutional framework.

Pre- and Post-SBM: Evidence from Across the Country

As an integral part of the programme, every batch of students at the Institute of Rural Management Anand (IRMA) participates in the Village Fieldwork Segment

(VFS), which includes an eight-week stay in the village in one of the households. The Village Fieldwork Segment (VFS) is conducted after the first classroom term, where they are taught rural/participatory research methodology and have a good grounding in quantitative and qualitative techniques. The objective of the eight-week term is to develop in the participants a deeper understanding and sensitivity to rural communities' concerns and to help them identify inherent constraints and opportunities. They are attached to a local host organisation and placed in villages across India during this period. The students execute small action-oriented tasks related to the host organisation's area of work, known as the Rural Action Component (RAC). They also participate in collaborative research work with faculty members from IRMA through detailed surveys and thematic research. The students prepare the reports under the guidance of one of the faculty members. These reports carry deep insights into the village life on different aspects of rural life such as livelihoods, culture, society, education, health, etc. In recent years some of these village reports have also focused on sanitation. Our search of IRMA fieldwork reports generated 28 reports that also focused on the issues of sanitation and open defecation in rural areas. The reports cover 32 villages from across 11 significant states. It covered Himachal Pradesh, Uttarakhand, and Uttar Pradesh from North India; Andhra Pradesh, Kerala, and Karnataka from South India; Gujarat and Rajasthan from Western India; and Bihar and Odisha from Eastern India. The reports cover a period from 2005 to 2017. Thus, the reports cover the pre-SBM and post-SBM periods.

During their eight-week village stay, the students use several methods and techniques to understand the rural reality. To obtain information, students use various participatory rural appraisal (PRA) techniques – historical timeline, resource map, social map, Venn (Chapati) diagram, household surveys, semi-structured interviews, and informal interactions and unobtrusive observations. They also conducted focus group discussions (FGDs) with villagers. They stayed in the village for about six to seven weeks, which allowed them to develop a strong rapport with the villagers. It was facilitated by the fact that they were staying in the house of one of the villagers, making them readily acceptable to the village community. Many of the insights were obtained through informal interactions.

Pre-SBM Stage

Arun Kumar had spent the autumn of 2005 in the village of Chotanala in the Kantharya Panchayat of the Jharol tehsil of the Udaipur district of Rajasthan. This village, located in the southern range of the Aravallis, falls into the Jharol Taluka of the Udaipur district. The majority of the present-day residents of the village hail from northern Gujarat and belong to the Gameti Bhil tribe. Like most tribal villages, it does not have a caste hierarchy. The community has unique water-sharing norms, with all the community members enjoying open and equal access to drinking, domestic, and cattle needs. However, an irrigation facility is available only to the individual owner of the well, while no irrigation needs are met from the community wells. Many wells are jointly owned, and here, the water for drinking and domestic needs is open to all while shared for irrigation purposes by the joint owners of the well. Many check dams have been constructed and trenches dug in the protected forest area. These are maintained by the community and repaired through free labour (*Shramdaan*) by a single member from each household. However, large-scale work such as de-siltation involves capital disbursed on demand by the Panchayat. Open defecation is the norm due to the complete absence of toilets in the village. Most people prefer the nearby stream area for open defecation. Additionally, the villagers use the stream water for washing clothes, cleaning utensils, bathing, and feeding cattle around the wells, which has led to groundwater contamination. The groundwater in the villages has more *E. Coli* content than that found in the sewage water of Udaipur city.

In 2008 from October through December, Ravi Kumar Dhanuka spent eight weeks understanding the rural life in Pranti, a village in the district Muzaffarpur in Bihar. He observed that most villagers knew about the harmful effects of open defecation and roughly kinds of diseases caused by human excreta left in the open. The knowledge about dealing with diarrhoeal diseases, closely linked with sanitary and hygienic practices, was generally fair. They resort to effective treatment methods, such as the oral rehydration solution. They also knew they should cover their food and wash their hands before and after defecating. It was found talking to the villagers that gradually, their attitude towards sanitation is shifting to the positive side from hostile or apathetic. He observed that the availability of toilets at home strengthened the householder's social status. It may be because the village is Muslim dominated in terms of population, and Muslims are more conservative in sending females out in the open. All said they would not like to marry their daughter to someone who did not have a toilet. No one appreciates the practice of going out for open defecation. It may be related to the perceived status of having toilets at home. Around 98%–99% of the respondents agreed that toilets at home strengthen the social status of the household. They believed those who go in the open are either shameless people or not left with any other option. According to them, no rational people would prefer going outside given the option. Ravi interviewed about 100 villagers; 98 considered using toilets economically beneficial in the long run. They considered the loss of workdays due to illnesses and the costs of medical treatment, environmental damage from the uncontrolled discharge of untreated wastes in and around urban areas, and the insecurity and risk of violence faced by women and children are the significant ill effects of open defecation. The villagers generally believed that open defecation bothered them a lot, making the place dirt and the foul smell intolerable. They said they pity those who cannot build toilets and curse those who do not build toilets. The thought that human excreta in the open does not portray a good image of the village adds to their worry. 'The eminent personalities will not enter my village if they see a toilet on the road', laments Nazima Khatun, a widow who works hard to feed herself and her ten children.

In a problem ranking exercise, where villagers are asked to rank the problems in the village, sanitation emerged as a significant problem. In one household survey, all respondents said they would not like to marry a daughter in a house that did not have a toilet. They also unequivocally said that not having toilets at home weakens their social status, and open defecation is distressful. However, on closer examination, many households in the village did not have toilet facilities at home. Out of approximately 950 households, 350 households had toilets, and only 267 toilets were functional. Secondly, out of these 267 toilets, 150 are not used by all household members. In an average family size of ten, one toilet does not suffice in the morning.

Moreover, many Muslim families prefer separate toilets for males and females. Therefore, males sometimes compromise because of congestion or not having a separate toilet. Across the age groups, youth are the most frequent users. Older people sometimes compromise with the excuse that it does not make much of a difference to them as they are used to it. Children aged 0–6 years care the least due to these aberrations present within the family. About 57% of the respondents said it had also been challenging for parents to teach good sanitation practices to children. However, every respondent household is used to washing hands with ash, soil, or soap after finishing their business in the toilet.

Some toilets were non-functional because some households (about 120) had an Ecosan model. The Ecosan model is promoted as eco-friendly because it does not require water and is a viable alternative to flush toilets in water-deficient areas. However, where the water table is high, the risk of groundwater contamination increases. There are usually two pits; when one pit of an Ecosan toilet fills up, it is sealed for about nine months. The compost is used as organic manure on the farms. Villagers are still not very comfortable with this new concept of pouring ash over excreta in place of water. Some owners did not follow the instructions for using this unique model, which invited stinking germs. Many are sceptical of using this model, thinking that their groundwater might also get affected, which is not misplaced as the water table in North Bihar is very high. It was also found that 70% of the older respondents were not particular about using toilets. It was not that they were obsessed with their habit of going out, but they did not put much effort into going to the toilet, especially when it came to urinating. Part of the reason is also attributed to the rural lifestyle. Many leave their home early for farmland. Children play naked in the open ground, defecating at the place they wish after being influenced by children who do not have toilets. Female farmworkers cannot look after the hygienic practices of their children as, most of the time, they are out to earn money. Few households in the village had built toilets for their guests; they seldom use them and thus have little motivation to keep them functional. It was also observed that when many villagers were without toilets, the members who had toilets may stop using toilets because of the urge to conform to the social norms.

During the interactions, many villagers contemplated breaking their toilets. There were some instances of breaking built-in toilets in the village. The places where water is very scarcely available, women broke toilets to prevent themselves from the drudgery of fetching water from long distances. One person broke the toilet because he was not happy with the model. However, this may be very few cases. But few cases can give us insights into the possible risks that one faces for a hundred percent defecation-free environment. One of the reasons for breaking the toilet may be because the opportunity cost of having a toilet is meagre.

Moreover, in this village, almost every household has a hand pump. Therefore, water is not an issue. However, one more concern is, will this large-scale shift in behaviour be sustainable and the toilets constructed will be maintained without any further interventions? Further, there is a kind of social control building up. In the village environment, dignity is much sought after, and as our results show, many people believe that toilets add to their social status. Thus, we can safely hope for the desirable result of sustainable behaviour and maintenance of toilets. The demand for toilets is the function of land, income, and awareness. Those who do not have a toilet cannot build their toilet no matter how much they desire it. The second important thing is income. Some people struggle to get a square meal. It is tough for them to save and incur expenses for maintaining the toilet.

Abhishek, Priyanka, and Subhradip spent about eight weeks in three different villages across two states (Himachal Pradesh and Odisha) during the village fieldwork segment in 2011. The three village studies, Tarda and Gunthuli in the Rayagada district of Odisha and Gangodi in the Solan district of Himachal Pradesh, threw up some exciting facts. Both Tarda and Gunthuli are located in the Eastern Ghats and are surrounded by hills and forests. Gangodi is located in the hilly terrains of the Solan district. Tarda Gram Vikas, an NGO in southern Odisha, has implemented the Total Sanitation Programme (TSP). They had constructed water tanks and supplied clean drinking water to the doorstep of every household in the village to improve the hygiene and sanitary condition in the village. They also constructed toilets and bathrooms for every individual household. These interventions have undoubtedly contributed to the improvement of the environmental hygiene of the village. As far as hygiene is considered, Tarda was considered a model village in the Panchayat. The Gunthuli village was in stark contrast to Tarda village. The sanitary conditions had significantly improved after implementing the TSP in Tarda. Every household had its bathrooms and toilets connected with a round-the-clock water supply. The NGO Gram Vikas constructed these. Hence, open defecation was a rare sight in the village. The teachings in the church also significantly influenced the sanitary condition of the village. They were made aware of various day-to-day hygienic practices in the church.

Unlike Tarda, TSP was not implemented in Gunthuli. Only a single person in the village had bathrooms and toilets attached to his home. Open defecation was a common preference among the villagers. People rarely used soaps after defecation and rarely washed their hands before eating. The cowsheds were near the living areas, further degrading the hygiene status in the village. The villagers bathed around the common wells in the village. These places did not have proper drainage systems, resulting in the waterlogging around them, providing a perfect condition for breeding malaria mosquitoes. The poor hygienic condition was reflected in the poor health status maintained by the villagers. A problem which was very common in Gangodi was regarding open defecation. Various awareness camps were organised in this regard. Disposal of waste is the main issue under hygiene. Like Tarda, there is the intervention of an NGO in this village.

There was an intervention of Gram Vikas in Tarda, due to which the villagers could have access to clean drinking water and closed bathrooms and toilets. The direct effect was visible in reducing the number of diseases in the village. Although it did not affect malaria, the effect on skin diseases was quite evident. The incidence of waterborne diseases had also come down. The difference was quite visible in the case of Gunthuli, which was devoid of NGO intervention. The incidence of malaria, skin diseases, and waterborne diseases was relatively high. The case of open defecation was utterly absent in Tarda, whereas it was a common practice in Gunthuli. As far as Gangodi was concerned, it had some similarities to Tarda. After the NGO intervention, people could use clean drinking water by administering chlorine water in the water tanks. The awareness regarding health and sanitation in the village increased.

In the Baletha village at Akbarpur Block in district Ramabai Nagar of Uttar Pradesh, Gurpreet Singh Chabbra spent eight weeks during the village fieldwork segment of 2011. He found that the sanitation facilities in the village are not very good. The overall awareness level of people regarding sanitation in the village was poor. People did not consider the toilet essential and did not figure it on their priority list. According to them, it does not matter much whether they go to toilets or open fields for excretion, and there is little connection between health and sanitation. A survey of about 40 households revealed that only about 12 households out of those 40 had toilet facilities.

Interestingly, out of the 12 households with toilets, all members were not using the toilet. Generally, the male family members will go out for open defecation. The toilets were connected to the septic tank. Most toilets in the village did not have doors, and a sari or any other cloth was used to cover them. Toilets, in many cases, were constructed behind the house because there was some social stigma still prevailing regarding toilets being constructed inside the households. A curious fact emerged: those with city relatives had constructed toilets in their village homes. Because when the relatives visited the village, they found it uncomfortable visiting fields for open defecation.

As per awareness and access to toilets, there was a class and caste divide in the village. Members of the upper caste who were also relatively affluent had greater awareness regarding sanitation. Even under government schemes of toilet construction, the upper caste people first applied for these schemes. Although sanitation facilities figured low in the priority list of upper and lower caste people, the condition was worse in lower caste groups. One reason was also the economic backwardness of these people. According to them, they were having problems earning two meals a day, so they were not concerned about whether there was a toilet at home or not. On the other hand, the upper caste people were relatively well-off (they could afford to construct and maintain toilets); they had relatives living in cities, so they were much more aware of clean sanitation facilities.

During the same year, Kireet Pande and Raja Panchal spent their fieldwork segment in two villages (Dora and Bhogpur) in the Solan district of Himachal Pradesh. They found that the Total Sanitation Campaign (TSC) launched by the Government of India had brought about a change among the people. The villagers are now building toilets and washrooms in their homes. However, this was achieved because of the harsh measures adopted by the government functionaries.

The household was denied the PDS benefits if they did not construct toilets in their homes. It positively impacted the villagers, and their attitude toward sanitation was changed. Toilets and washrooms have encouraged cleanliness and good health. The development of toilets has been of particular benefit for the women of the village, who now no longer have to make hazardous trips to the fields after dark. Washrooms are also giving them a feeling of privacy. The measures are expected to help improve the villagers' health status in the long run. The presence of toilets has also improved the village's cleanliness and sanitary conditions as the villagers no longer defecate in the open.

The village fieldwork report of Prateek Parimal, who had spent eight weeks in Sharfuddinpur village in the Muzaffarpur district of Bihar in 2011, suggested that despite the relatively better infrastructural condition of the village relative to other villages in the district, the quality of facilities in terms of basic amenities like drinking water and sanitation was still poor. There has been a shift in the economic and social condition of the villagers in the last couple of years, yet the awareness level of the villagers is still very low. They stated they had the opportunity to talk to many villagers, about 50 households out of over 300 households in the village with their tube well and separate toilets. Despite the relatively high groundwater level in these areas, one can get water at about 50 feet deep; the rest of the villagers had poor drinking water and sanitation conditions. However, there was a precise cut class and caste divide regarding access to sanitation and water. The village is comprised of four tolas or hamlets. The hamlets are segregated in terms of religious and caste lines.

The Choudhary tola, the most prosperous neighbourhood in the village, comprised Choudhary, who belonged to the landowning castes. It was the most prosperous hamlet present in the village regarding the resources available to the people living there. There was not a single makeshift (kaccha) household in that hamlet, and even there were three-storied pucca houses. Each household has a hand pump and a toilet facility that was not shared with other households. Some houses even have a well-built separate toilet situated far from the drinking water source in the house. The residents of this hamlet were well aware of the sanitation needs.

There was another hamlet which was exclusively inhabited by Muslims – Muslim tola. This hamlet was situated at one corner of the village and had quite a different social and infrastructural facility than the rest. Although some houses have got their hand pumps, this hamlet's health-seeking aspect was deficient. Most of the houses have only pit toilets which were not well maintained, and the people used to go to open fields to defecate. The Dhobi tola hamlet was situated near the Chaudhary tola and was relatively prosperous. Some houses have built artificial water tanks in front of their houses, used to wash clothes. All houses have hand pumps used for washing clothes. All the houses in this hamlet were relatively well built and had toilets, which were not shared with other households. Mushahar tola residents were at the bottom of the social hierarchy; they were cut off from the rest of the village and were located at one end of the village. A *Kaccha* road connected this hamlet with the main village, and drinking water and sanitation conditions were deplorable. There were only 5 hand pumps for 45 households, and 2 of them were not functioning well. There were no drains in the hamlet. Only three houses owned a toilet built with the Gram Panchayat; otherwise, the rest of the households were forced to go for open defecation. Thus, the water and sanitation facilities in this hamlet were the worst. People had low awareness levels, which prevented them from availing better services from the government's existing schemes.

At the village level, no such interventions could be sighted in terms of any example for drinking water or environmental sanitation by the community. There is no drainage system for the wastewater flowing from the houses. When the student asked why they were not constructing toilets when the government scheme for construction existed, they responded, 'what is the benefit of constructing the toilet? As long as we have our agricultural fields, we can go there; there is no point in wasting our hard-earned money. Toilets are meant for rich people.'

During the fieldwork segment of 2011, Abhishek Sharma spent his weeks studying the Chimana village in the Bikaner district of Rajasthan. The Chimana village is located in the Thar desert of Rajasthan, an arid area in stark contrast to the high water table areas of Muzaffarpur of Bihar. However, the contrast ends here. In this village, only ten households had toilets. Dunes surround the village. The most precious thing in the village is water. The water used by the villagers is highly saline. According to the PHED junior engineer, the fluoride contents are high in the water. The quality of water is seldom monitored, and the kits given by the department are relatively unused. Since most village inhabitants consume water from tube wells, water quality is the same across all the social groups. The majority of people in the village defecate in the open. Those who can afford toilets also do not make it as they find it a wasteful expenditure. One of the few homes in the village has a toilet. Most of the people live in their fields called 'Dhanis'. So there is no one particular place to defecate. Four tube wells in the village were managed by the Public Health and Engineering Department (of the government of Rajasthan), and Gram Panchayat manages another one. There hasn't been much development on this front. PHED has kept water monitoring kits in the Panchayat to monitor water quality. In the sanitation segment, there was one scheme through which villagers were given Rs. 3200 to construct toilets. But according to the Sarpanch, Rs. 3200 is not enough to construct toilets, so nobody asks for the money. Secondly, due to the unavailability of water, people think toilets will put an extra burden on fetching water.

In 2012, Parnika Tripathi went for her fieldwork in the Bhutardi village of the Dahod district of Gujarat. The village was located on the banks of river Dudhimati. The entire village had only three households with a toilet in their homes. Barring these three households, the entire village preferred open defecation. Through informal interactions, the villagers were careful not to defecate near the water sources as they knew the potential health threats it could lead to. When asked how far they walked from their respective houses to the point of defection, they replied that it was rarely fixed and generally in the walking range of 15 minutes. Many of them preferred to defecate on their farms as it saved them from the embarrassment of being caught. A common notion among the villagers was that toilets within the premises caused diseases, and defecating on the farms was far more hygienic than using a toilet. They only realised the essence of a toilet when they suffered from loose motions because they all suffered severe privacy issues. Another challenge in having toilets at home was water scarcity. Women of the household usually fetch water. The data provided by women on time spent fetching water suggested that they spent about one hour every day just fetching drinking water. Every family fetched water twice a day, i.e., morning and evening. Mostly women and children below 18 years went to fetch water from the well. Thus, many women opposed the idea of toilets at home, fearing a more significant workload for them.

Amit Kumar spent the fieldwork of 2012 in Pandutalab village located in the foothills of Malwa plateau in Dewas district of Madhya Pradesh. This area is close to Omkareshwar, famous for the Jyotirlinga of Lord Shiva, and Indore, which is just 60 km away. In contrast to the Rajasthan and Gujarat villages, this village had an excellent rainfall of about 750–1100 mm on average. The majority (about 78%) of villagers are from tribal communities. The village has poor sanitation services in general. Only a few households (less than eight) have toilets.

Moreover, this trend is across the community irrespective of economic well-being and social status. People who can afford the toilets also do not build them partly because of a lack of awareness and poverty. The villagers feel that space is never a constraint, so there is no urge to build a toilet. In addition, due to living in fields, there is no particular place for defecation and defecation in the open has not created many problems of cleanliness in the area. Toilets constructed in the villages are of two types. The economically well-off section – the Jaiswal, which constituted very few households – have constructed toilets in their homes at their own expense. The tribal households below the poverty line group built the toilets under the Indira Awas Yojana or the Total Sanitation Campaign (TCS). Apart from this, a small number of tribal households had toilets due to NGO awareness; most were working with them at some point. Another trend emerging among those who used to migrate to the upper Malwa plateau and nearby towns is their willingness to construct a toilet. They are in the mood to even invest some money in constructing a toilet if the government supports a little more than what they can personally contribute now.

Even if the family has a toilet, most members do not use that facility. The chief reason for the non-use of toilets was the low quality of construction, shortage of water, and apprehension that toilets would make their house dirty. Secondly, many in the village thought there were enough open spaces to defecate. One villager said, ‘there are enough open spaces in and around our village, so why should we waste money, time, and space constructing a toilet?’ Another lady added, ‘it will lead to the additional burden of bringing more water from the water source for the toilet; we will have to do all the dirty work of cleaning the toilet. Construction of toilets will only make us do the donkey’s work.’ In the houses that had constructed toilets, the responsibility for cleaning toilets rested with the women. People also said the subsidy amount provided for the construction of toilets was insufficient. Secondly, there were worries about the pit becoming full at some point. It seemed that the two-pit system was not in the design element for building toilets at that time.

During the discussions with children, parents, and teachers, the demand for a toilet at school did not emerge as a concern – this was as if not having a toilet in school was the most natural thing to happen. Similarly, at the Anganwadi centres, there was no concern for toilets. None of the women mentioned the need for having a toilet at the Anganwadi centre. On questions about hygiene, a relatively good level of understanding was present among the children regarding various aspects of personal hygiene, including knowledge about waterborne diseases, the importance of handwashing, brushing teeth, taking regular baths, and how to treat water. They also knew about the negative effect of open defecation. Despite such understanding, there was a wide gap as far as the practices were concerned. The houses that have constructed toilets on their premises have a constant foul smell.

Manish Gautam and Tonmoie Sarmah spent their fieldwork during the autumn of 2012 in the Bari and Bhadsin villages, respectively, part of the Bilaspur district of Himachal Pradesh. Bhadsin was a small village comprising 30 households. The households were spread within a land area of about 20 acres. The village mainly consisted of two castes, i.e., Brahmins and Khatris. Twenty-eight households out of the total were Brahmins, and only two households belonged to the Khatris.

On the other hand, the village Bari had 114 households. Bari was subdivided into Bari Kalan and Bari Khurd. The total area of the village is 137.5 acres. Thus, the two villages provided a contrast in terms of size. Despite the differences in size, the villages were at the forefront of the sanitation movement. Due to the positive steps taken by the Government of Himachal Pradesh, many villages in the state saw a drastic improvement in sanitation. Both the Panchayats had received Nirmal Gram Puraskar in 2008. Every household in the village of Bhadsin had a personal toilet, so no cases of open defecation were reported. People in both the villages were aware and conscious of having a toilet facility at home.

A lot of importance was given to women's security, one reason for having toilets at home. Thus, the Total Sanitation Campaign (TCS) was implemented effectively in both the villages. TSC has played a significant role in supporting and creating awareness among the villagers. Ventilated improved pit toilets were seen in both the villages. Toilets were pucca, and no *kuccha* (non-permanent structure) toilets were seen. A ventilated improved pit toilet is a dry pit toilet. A ventilator pipe is attached to it behind the toilet and reaches above the roof of the toilet. The mouth of the pipe is covered with a wire mesh or a net to prevent flies and other insects, including dry leaves of trees, from getting into it. The pipe helps in keeping the foul smell out. Few households in the villages were seen to be having Western-style toilets also. Funds were provided under MGNREGA and TSC for the construction of toilets. Villagers in both the villages were economically not so poor, so only a few families relied on the funds for the construction of toilets. In villages, pits were constructed below or back of the toilet. The problem of the pit getting chocked was resolved by cementing all the four sides of the pit except the base. Guests accommodated in others' homes were allowed to use their toilets.

The village fieldwork report presented by Priyanka Mehta in 2012 reported her experience of fieldwork in the village Govindsar, about 70 km from the international border with Pakistan, located in Bikaner district in the northwestern part of

Rajasthan. The area falls under an arid zone and receives an average annual rainfall of 12–25 cm. Under the Indira Gandhi Nahar Pariyojana (IGNP), the canal flows through the area. In the rainy season, extra water from the canal is released to a water reservoir close to 10 square km in area. This lake is called the Manori Talai, which forms the main water reservoir for the village. There were about 300 households in the village. In the entire village, only 13 households had built-in toilets. The toilets were also a symbol of the economic prosperity of the household. The rest of the households practised open defecation.

Ravi Kumar Yadav spent his 2012 fieldwork segment in Dahinda village of Burhanpur district of Madhya Pradesh. Earlier, the village was part of the Khandwa district, but due to one village's submerging, the village's administration was transferred to Burhanpur. It is equidistant from both Khandwa and Burhanpur districts and well connected to them through a state highway, which connects them. It is a revenue village. It falls under Dahinda Gram Panchayat. It is a tribal village, and the people are of the Korku tribe. Open defecation has been the norm in the village. Only 10 households from among 400 households had toilets; all of these toilets were privately built. During the fieldwork, the Village Panchayat constructed two model toilets using government funds. During 2007–8 kutcha toilets were constructed for BPL households under a total sanitation campaign for Rs. 1200 per toilet. These comprised the seat, surrounded by bamboo walls and an asbestos roof. Each toilet cost around Rs. 10000 and was jointly funded by TSC, NREGA, and some amount was paid by the beneficiary. Thus, almost all go for open defecation. However, a positive change is taking place. With the sensitisation programme carried out by AKRS(I), many women from the village are coming forward to demand toilets. During the fieldwork, 60 applications were received for availing toilet facility at home.

During the 2012 fieldwork segment, Surbhi Sood lived for about eight weeks in Kojawara village, situated in the southern district of Rajasthan known as Udaipur. It is located at a distance of 80 km from the city of Udaipur, and the nearest towns are Rishabhdev and Kherwara at a distance of 15 km and 16 km from the village, respectively. It comes under the Kojawara Panchayat with two other villages, Pareda Jagir and Parada Chak. The Panchayat is located at Kherwara, whereas the village comes under the Rishabhdev tehsil. The village is spread over 1982 hectares and has a population of 3081, of which 49% are females and 70% belong to the scheduled tribe such as the Meena tribe (as of 2001 census). As the village lies in the Aravalli hill ranges, the terrain is mostly rocky and undulating, with some plain land. There are 522 households in the village, mainly belonging to castes such as Patel, Meena, Kalal, and Meghwal. A predominantly tribal village, the population consists mainly of Meena and Patel castes. Out of the 522 households, 31 households have toilet facilities. Most villagers, including a few who have toilets at home, defecate in the open. Incidentally, 20 households did not use the toilets because of various reasons. A short survey revealed the following reasons for not using the toilets at home.

Many of the toilets and bathrooms constructed are not being used. Common reasons for the same are as follows:

An open defecation is a form of social gathering.
There is difficulty in changing lifelong habits.
Toilet has alternative uses like store rooms for grain, tethering goats, etc.
There is difficulty in maintaining toilet at home.
A toilet is meant only for women members of the household.
The financial aid being given currently to the villagers is not enough.

On further investigation, it was found that most toilets were not in working conditions due to faulty design and construction, and the pit toilet becoming full is another cause. However, in most cases, the overwhelming explanation for not using the toilet was the habit of open defecation and social pressure.

Utsav Agarwal studied the sanitation conditions of village Tholapalli in the Chikballapur district of Karnataka in 2012. There are 171 households in the village and several institutions like Anganwadis, schools, Panchayat, fair price shops, etc. So there is a requirement of approximately 200 toilets in the village after counting the community toilets that must be located strategically. The village sadly has only two toilets in working conditions. The government has launched several schemes which gave a grant of Rs. 9000 for the construction of each toilet. However, extremely substandard work is done, and the government subsidy is shared between the beneficiary and officials. Thus, the toilets constructed per government records are never used for their intended purpose but as a storage facility by the households. Some have not even bothered to construct any structure and spent the money. The government stipulates the requirement of an overhead water tank for piped water supply to every household. Still, none of the households of the hamlets of Manda and the Ambedkar Colony has it. Flush toilets are useless if the residents don't have piped water supply. The area has rocky terrain, and the construction of a safety tank is also tricky. Another reason for government schemes' failure is the water scarcity in the region. The student explored the construction of community toilets in the village.

No nodal agency or NGO is working on sanitation in this village. IRMA students contacted several agencies, including Mr Paul Calvert, India's leading authority on Ecosan toilets. At the same time, they explored the possibility of having Ecosan toilets in the village with very little water availability. A focus group discussion (FGD with the village threw up several issues. Still, most notably, the underlying message was that the women were not enthusiastic about having toilets at home. Later, Mr Paul Calvert said that if the community refuses to accept the project, it is sure to fail. He cited several instances where Ecosan toilets resemble ghost structures because the community was not taken into confidence. Thus, the norm of open defecation continued.

During the same time, the report by Megha Choudhry from the village of Koruwa in Dehradun district of Uttarakhand (fieldwork of 2012) was different from the one received from the village in Karnataka. The village was a typical tribal village in the Jaunsar-Bawar region. This whole belt was declared tribal by the government in 1966. Situated at around 7249 feet the region is bordered by river Yamuna in the east and river Tons in the west. Parts of Uttarkashi define the northern boundary, and Himachal Pradesh and Dehradun lie to its south. It is 10 km away from the Chakrata army base camp, which was earlier the cantonment area of the Britishers. It comes under Atal Adarsh Gram. The nearest town is Vikasnagar which is 30 km away.

The condition of sanitation facilities in Koruwa is good. Most of the households had toilets in their dwellings. The types of toilets present were pit toilets with a slab. Many of the toilets were made under Nirmal Bharat Abhiyan; they had benefitted the BPL families. They had awareness regarding good sanitation facilities. They considered it essential to have toilets in their houses not just as a social status but a necessity. People had used the government incentive of Rs. 2700 to make toilets. The families who did not have toilets were mainly the poor Harijan families who could not afford to make toilets. The estimated expense of making a toilet is about Rs. 15000 in this region because it is located at a high altitude and the terrain is a difficult therefore, lot of effort is needed to move materials from the plains, which increases the cost of construction. The families who had toilets used buckets to flush or had taps in the toilets themselves. These families used ashes as well as soap to wash their hands. The toilets had ventilation as well as doors. Only the toilets constructed recently did not have doors. All the members of the house used the toilet facility. No community sanitation complexes were present in the village, and sharing toilets between two or more families was also not done. But there was one strange practice where the waste of infants was not disposed of into the toilets but was washed down the hills with water. The primary school, secondary school, Anganwadi, as well as Kasturba Gandhi Balika Vidyalaya also had their functional toilets.

There was a difference across the tribal groups and caste groups in the construction and use of the toilets. Koruwa had people of scheduled tribes and scheduled caste. The majority were of scheduled tribes and were also more affluent than people of scheduled caste. The awareness regarding using sanitation facilities was almost equal with different castes. But the people of the scheduled caste, being poor, could not afford to get toilets constructed because of financial reasons. They said that the money government gave was not enough to construct the toilet. Many families had Rs. 2700 to make toilets, but the family consumed this money. One reason was also the economic backwardness of these people. According to them, they had problems earning two meals a day, so they were not concerned about whether they had a toilet facility in their homes.

Post-SBM Stage

In 2015 Ankita Jain and Shivani Lochab prepared a report based on their eight-week extended stay in the Suryanarayanpur village of Ganjam district in Odisha. Suryanarayanpur has 142 households and a total population of 791. Before 2002, the villagers defecated in the open. It led to increased diarrhoea and other water-borne diseases in the village. After the intervention by Gram Vikas, only 10 households out of 142 did not have proper sanitation facilities. But it was observed that women defecate in the open during menstruation. Personal hygiene is not taken seriously during that time. The elder also defecates in the open. It is because they are accustomed to the old habits and find it very difficult to use toilets. Ankita conducted several interviews with the villagers to understand the status of sanitation in Suryanarayanpur.

The Case of Nillama

Nillama – 'It's a Women Issue' Nillama, 40 years, is an important member of the village water committee. In 2002, she helped Gram Vikas staff to encourage the villagers to construct toilets. On asking about how frequently she uses the toilet, she replied that she never uses the toilet during menstruation. She feels that the house will become dirty, and the goddess of wealth will refuse to bless their house. She is educated till the eighth standard, and she works with Anganwadi as a helper. She has been trained by the Orissa government on issues like women's health and menstruation; still, she prefers to lose her sanity than protesting for the issues. She said that a menstruating woman generally goes to the pond or on the outskirt of the village to defecate. This has been a custom for generations and has been followed blindly. Nobody has complained of inconvenience from this system. The elders in the family are the main decision-makers. Women are more conservative, and they go to defecate outside either early morning or late at night. She has suffered from diarrhoea twice in this year.

The Case of Pillisimadri

Pillisimadri is 62 years old and suffering from elephantiasis, a parasitic infection causing swelling of both arms and legs. The disease is caused by the transmission from one person to the other through a female mosquito. He described that before 2002, the sanitation conditions were terrible in the village. There was a malaria and diarrhoea outbreak now and then. Any outsider who came to the village used to turn up their noses because the village's periphery was loaded with human faeces. He was getting treated for this disease. He said that his health expenditures have increased from the past three years to Rs. 1500. There are five ponds in the village. They were the primary water source before the Gram Vikas water tank came in. This water was used for domestic as well as drinking purposes. Community members used to defecate in those ponds. He believed that Gram Vikas's intervention proved to be helpful for the village because it was not only about toilets but also about dignity. He considers open defecation acceptable for children and elders. Every year two of his family members suffer from diarrhoea. His mother suffered from diarrhoea for a year almost. He discards the fact that the building of toilets is linked with hygiene. He feels that the need for water motivated him and the villagers to build toilets. Hygiene is a secondary issue to his family.

Gram Vikas, the NGO operating in this area, has taken up the task of raising awareness about health and hygiene in southern Odisha. It, through constant interaction with the villagers, has motivated the villagers, who are mostly from tribal communities, to construct toilets. In order to maintain and sustain the system, it has encouraged the villagers to construct overhead water tanks in each village which is connected through pipe to each household. Gram Vikas, from the initial years, has steadfastly argued for 100% inclusion of all households in the sanitation programme. The necessity of this is driven home in the argument that the waste disposal behaviour of a single household is likely to affect the quality of drinking water for the entire community. Once the community agrees to the 100% norm, collecting materials and formalising the roles and responsibilities of the Village Executive committee start. The village-level executive committee, comprising 50% women, takes charge of the entire water supply system, its operations, and running expenses with proper utilisation of the water bill collected every month. It is the key to project sustainability after Gram Vikas exits the village. One of the significant departures of the Gram Vikas model is that a bathroom is attached to the toilet. The toilet is not designed as a cubbyhole where you leave the excreta but rather a place to clean yourself. Attaching the bathroom has a significant implication in people's efforts to clean the place. For women, the bathroom attached to the toilet has a greater significance than ordinarily thought and discussed. In a standalone toilet, the women experience privacy and safety. However, in the absence of a bathroom, they will come out in the open, take a bath, and clean themselves in the open, i.e., on riverbanks, ponds, or just near the well. Bathing in the open is as severe a threat to safety as open defecation. Secondly, the element of shame is discomforting for them and often becomes a cause of shame and endangers their security.

Each household in the village will construct a toilet with a bathroom. Communities and staff are trained to monitor water quality. Some measures include regular cleaning of water tanks and chlorination of water sources to control bacteriological contamination during heavy downpours. Through monetary contribution and active participation in construction, communities contribute towards the cost of development and maintenance of facilities. On an average each family contributes 60% of the cost of sanitation and bathing infrastructure and 30% of the cost of establishing a piped water supply system. Each village also mobilises a 'corpus fund' that is a one-time collection raised through an average contribution of Rs. 1000 per household. This fund is placed in a term deposit in a bank. Using the interest of the corpus funds new families in the villages are supported to build their sanitation facilities after Gram Vikas has withdrawn from the village. Hygiene and sanitation education and building toilets and bathing rooms are half the battle in improving health conditions of the rural communities. Therefore efforts are made to intensify education on hygiene practices. The link between diseases and hand washing with soaps is emphasised. Staff also educate on environment cleanliness and carry out village cleanliness drives.

Privacy and Dignity of Women

Earlier women used to wait for the specific time of the day to do their daily work like cleaning, bathing, etc. They suffered from lack of privacy and safety as it was not always safe to go out to nearby ponds and fields. There were many incidences of insect bites and molestation. With the construction of bathing rooms and toilets now women are free from privacy and safety concerns. Still because of some traditional taboos females were not allowed to use household toilets, and they had to go out for defecation. This remains the bottleneck in the successful implementation of the entire programme. It hampers the idea of improving hygiene practices and health status. Also some girls dispose of sanitary pads in the ponds which further pollutes water resources.

Sheel Bhadra, another participant of the postgraduate programme, did his fieldwork in another village in the same district during 2016. His village was Kanamana. Kanamana (pronounced 'Konamona') is a village situated in Chhatrapur block of Ganjam district in the state of Odisha. It is located about three kilometres west of Gopalpur port which lies along the beach of Bay of Bengal. Kanamana can be accessed via rail and road. The nearest railway station is Chhatrapur (station code : CAP), which is four kilometres west of the village. Autorickshaws ply on a regular basis to and from Chhatrapur. Kanamana is a revenue village and comes under the Kanamana Panchayat which comprises six villages including Kanamana and its hamlet, Chasa Kanamana. The sanitation programme has led to an end to open defecation. The villagers earlier used to go to the fields or the nearby ponds, etc., to defecate but now since they have toilets constructed within their homes, they do not need to go out. Since they also have a bathroom it has become convenient, especially for the ladies, to take baths. Every household gets 24-hour water supply of potable water. Every household receives the same quality of water through pipelines that operate three taps per household – one in the kitchen, one in the bathroom, and one in the toilet. Since the water is good, potable groundwater and is further treated by chlorination before supply, no further boiling/purification is required before drinking it. People are satisfied with the quality and quantity supplied, and they do not need to go anywhere to fetch water to fulfil their requirements. Neither do they face any health-related problems by drinking this water. A walk of about one and a half kilometres twice a day to fetch water from the tube wells/ponds is not required anymore. The villagers are free to use the saved time the way they want. Some give more time to income-generating activities, some utilise this time to exercise, some are able to manage household chores more properly, and so on and so forth. Due to the impacts this programme has had on the village, the residents consider it to be of equal importance as Sri Venugopal Temple, which is the most important institution in the village.

In 2015 Rajshree Nancy was placed in the Pai village of Udaipur district in Rajasthan. There were 824 households in the village out of which 409 BPL families have received the monetary help of Rs. 12000 for the construction of toilets in their homes. About 60% of households have toilets but of those who have toilets many of them do not use them. The village is situated amidst the lush green hills of the Aravallis. Its scenic beauty is par excellence. It is surrounded by three ponds. It is a tribal village. The villagers provide several reasons for not using the toilets; the chief reasons are: water scarcity, badly designed and badly constructed toilets – not usable, improper water management, and lack of awareness on the implications of health. The people have been defecating in the open since birth, and this has become a practice for them. They do not know the implications that it can have on their health. The elders did not want to change their way of life at any cost whereas the younger generation was willing to embrace the change. The financial help provided by the government was also misused. They used it either for satisfying their grave personal needs or spent it on consuming alcohol. Some of them used only a portion of the money for construction of toilets. Hence they bought very poor-quality material that quickly broke away and became unusable. The Panchayat came up with a solution to this. They did not provide the entire amount of money to the beneficiaries. They instead provided them with all the construction material and paid only the labour charges. The people outsmarted them by selling the construction material and used the money for other purposes. Some toilets have been dilapidated because of their non-usage.

Jyoti Sharma in 2016 conducted the fieldwork in Khamhar village of Begusarai district in Bihar. Khamhar is a small village located to the north of Rajaura, eight kilometres from Begusarai city. Village Khamhar consists of ten wards and forms a part of Begusarai district of Bihar. The district lies on the northern bank of river Ganges. The survey results suggested that all villagers know about toilets and were aware of toilet construction schemes of SBM. They were aware of the amount provided by the government under the scheme but only 75% of people know about the complete paperwork that is required to be done to avail the benefits under the scheme. They were not aware of online forms available on the internet for the scheme. People were aware of only a few benefits of toilets like privacy and easy access. A survey of attitudes towards toilets revealed that people prefer toilets at home because of ease of access, when they are sick; it is good for the safety and security of women. A toilet at home is more comfortable for elderly people who are most vulnerable to injuries during night and rainy seasons. The area for open defecation is far and filthy. However, many villagers felt that open defecation gives them more pleasure and comfort. A toilet at home is suffocating; open defecation makes people early risers. They believed that they cannot eat and defecate under the same roof. Some villagers saw open defecation as an opportunity for socialisation. Also they believe that a single toilet cannot cater to the needs of the whole family. Most people in the village indicated that the main reason for not constructing a toilet is the cost. Other reasons for not owning a toilet include insufficient space and the resistance from elders about constructing a toilet.

Many households without a toilet understand and appreciate the benefits of a toilet but are too poor to afford it. While studying the costs of having a toilet in the village, the student was told by the village women that they would very much like to have toilets at home, but there is constant resistance from the elders in the household. To avoid conflict, they do not raise the issue of toilets at home. They are made to understand strictly the culture of their homes where their forefathers went to open fields to defecate, including their mother-in-law. They are made to understand that toilets are a waste of resources. Women face criticism when they go against their elders. They are looked down as women who do not respect their elders and wish to take control of the house. The neighbours do not respect these women, and hence women living in the neighbourhood do not invite these women to evening chit-chats out of fear of their respective elders. All these things affect the prestige of these women in society.

During her stay, she found that people were aware of the benefits of having toilets. A good social status and privacy were prime reasons for getting a toilet built in their homes. When asked about the economic cost of having toilets considering health, lifestyle, and water usage, most respondents pointed out that more water is used in toilets to keep those clean and odour free. People did not have water taps in their toilets. They fill water in buckets at hand pumps and carry them to the toilet, which increases their workload also. They have to spend a certain amount of money to buy acid to clean it. While interviewing people who do not own a toilet, she found the opportunity cost associated with having a toilet at home. Respondents shared that they could have invested their money in different things if they had not invested it in constructing toilets. Those different things include an android mobile set, LED television, a whitewash of their homes, and a stock of pesticides for their farm.

Case of Nigam Devi

Nigam Devi, 30 years old, stays in central Khamhar, belonging to the Bhumihaar caste. She has two daughters and a son. They finally got a toilet in their home a year back but had to pay a hefty social cost. She got a toilet at the cost of her family's integrity, respect, and prestige. Nigam Devi came to reside in Khamhar village after her marriage ten years back. There was no toilet in her new home, although she had one in her home before marriage. She had difficulty going out to defecate. The area was far away and filthy. She felt embarrassed there. She faced problems during the night or when she was not well. But she did not complain about it. However, she told her mother-in-law about the same, who refused to help her. She felt helpless, but her desire to own a toilet remained in her mind. During the intervening years, she gave birth to two daughters. After reaching pre-adolescent age, her elder daughter started complaining about the problems she faced while defecating in the open. Nigam did not want her daughter to feel embarrassed and ashamed, which she had felt throughout her existence in Khamar village. That is when she resolved firmly to have a toilet at home. She put forward the proposal. But in-laws were against the construction of toilets. She was made to understand that toilets will lead to wastage of area and resources. She was even abused. But she did not give up. Over time, she successfully persuaded her husband but failed to pursue her in-laws. There were fights in the house, which gradually became the order of the day. The situation went out of control and finally led to partition. Now the in-laws live in a separate house. They do not talk to her and her daughters. There was a sort of family-level ostracisation, coupled with her husband's regular taunts about how she had divided the family over a mere toilet.

The children missed their grandparents but did understand that the toilet at home gave them freedom and dignity. However, despite such trials and tribulations, she is happy as she feels that she did what was right and required. Thus, in the village, open defecation is not widely recognised as a health threat. They did not see the negative relationship between open defecation and children's health. Despite having a toilet at home, people who defecate cite pleasure and comfort as the prime reason. Many respondents indicated that open defecation is also an opportunity to get the fresh morning air and take morning walks. They believed that a single toilet could not cater to the whole family's needs.

In 2016 Rupal Bhargava studied the practice of open defecation in Kaparpura village of Muzaffarpur district of Bihar. The village had a mixed population of Hindus and Muslims. Hindus and Muslims have different settlements, but there are no conflicts. Among Hindus, there are nine social castes and occupational groups, and they live separately in different neighbourhoods, which are referred to as 'Tola'. These caste groups are mainly based on ancestral jobs performed by the respective groups such as Bhoomiyar tola, Baniya tola, Taili tola, Muslim Tola, Pasi tola, and Nooniya tola, Chamaar tola, Turha tola, and Refugee tola. In this village, open defecation is a common practice. There are no toilets constructed yet under the SBM scheme. When asked about it in the block office, we were told there was no budget allocation. People didn't know about the scheme.

People were not involved in deciding the type and structure of toilets they needed. The ring toilets constructed by the government have a high maintenance cost and no proper monitoring. There are various reasons for open defecation and lack of interest in constructing toilets, and the primary reason is poverty. For example, Laxmi Yadav, belonging to the Kurmi caste, is a poor woman without any agricultural land. She has a 12-member family. They had got a pit toilet constructed a few years back with the help of government funds. The pit got filled up, and they could not get it cleaned as cleaning the pit costs about Rs. 1500, which is prohibitively costly for them. So at present, all the family men go out in the open to avoid the early filling of the pit.

People did not feel the need to construct toilets. They did not see the health benefits they could get. The toilets were constructed based on perceived economic and social benefits. In another case, a Muslim family with 40 members in the house got a pit toilet constructed in 2004. They had paid Rs. 12000 for it. The family members believed the government looted them. They valued the toilet at Rs 5000 and felt cheated. Since people were not involved in the formulation of the scheme, the government lost faith in the public. Secondly, family size matters. Families with a large number of members suffer from a single toilet. Most male members go out to defecate in the open as there is only one toilet at home; most women use the toilet at home.

Caste and class divide within the village hinders the construction of community toilets., The people in the same community having different economic statuses will not contribute equally towards construction – this is where the community action has failed. Similarly, instances of cheating within the community have created the problem of trust. There was a movement to create a community toilet among the Pasi community. A leader from the community showed initiative; he was also a government official. He collected Rs 50 per family with signatures and made it look like the government would put in some money to construct toilets. Finally, the toilet was constructed, one for men and one for women; later, he constructed a wall around the toilets and blocked access of the same community members who had contributed to the construction of the toilet. Nobody except his family members was allowed to use it.

Cases of rapes, kidnapping, and molestation of girls were reported due to the open defecation in the village. But it was always pushed under the carpet, and women members were not allowed to speak about it. There was a case where an older woman constructed a toilet by mortgaging her jewellery. She once went out for the toilet in the dark. Later she realised she was defecating in the middle of snakes. Another problem in toilet construction in the village is that there are no well-defined property rights, particularly among members of large families. Secondly, certain sections of society do not have land ownership. These are landless migrants who had come to the village about some 20–30 years ago and settled on an abandoned old road. There was no opposition to it at that time as they supplied cheap labour to the village, particularly to the well-off farming families. However, they did not enjoy essential services like electricity and water supply. As they have no legal ownership of the land on which they are living and are waiting for the government to rehabilitate them, they are not in a position to invest in a toilet. Thus, a large section of the population will continue to defecate in the open.

Surbhi Jain conducted her fieldwork in the Shergarh village of the Jodhpur district of Rajasthan, located about 100 km west of the historic city of Jodhpur. Shergarh is a typical village in the Thar, dry and dusty, with a population of 6016 with over 1000 households; it can be considered a big village. Like many other villages in Shergarh, the work of SBM had started. Still, around 30% of total households do not have toilets at home or have no plans to construct them; 25% of the households have a toilet under construction, and the rest, 45%, have toilets at home, and about 10% of the completed toilets are not in working condition. Open defecation is largely present despite the availability of toilets. However, the available toilets are not used because they are either non-functional due to improper sanitary fitting and sewage systems or people consider it an unclean practice to go in closed spaces. Although toilets have been constructed under 'Swachh Bharat Abhiyan', people prefer open defecation because they are reluctant to change their age-old practices of going out for defecation in the open; they consider it unhygienic to go for defecation within the premises of their homes.

The reason for the open defecation of adolescent girls in APL households is the unacceptability of use of toilets within household premises. They do not consider building a toilet within household premises, as they believe that it will contaminate the food and water. In interviews with adolescent girls they expressed the unfortunate incidents they had to face because of open defecation. Even though all of them are aware of the ill effects of open defecation on their health and dignity, they cannot oppose it since they are not allowed in decision-making of household matters. Most of the adolescent girls prefer going for defecation either at dusk or at dawn so that they can do it hideously. Insects' bites while defecating are everyday miseries they go through. There have been some bigger mishaps like thefts, snake, and dog bites.

Case of Neelam

Neelam, a 17-year-old girl, recently got married to a construction worker. She belongs to the Bhil caste of the ST category. Neelam has big scars on her hand. After being enquired about the scar she narrated the unfortunate incident that happened with her when she was 13 years old. Four years ago, on a winter morning she went to a nearby barren land to defecate. She was alone as her mother was looking after the newborn in the family. Suddenly she was attacked by a fox hiding in the bushes. The fox pulled a piece of flesh from her right hand after which she had to undergo three months of treatment. The most unfortunate thing is that she still has to go for open defecation. She belongs to a BPL household. According to the family, constructing and maintaining a toilet is out of their budget. Although all schools have separate toilet facilities for girls and boys, as per survey, the toilets at school are not cleaned regularly. They are cleaned only previous to audits or inspections. Fortunately, the girls who stay in hostels have access to clean toilets as they are regularly cleaned.

Ebel Benny, Pravin Reddy, and Karan Garg studied sanitation practices in Chemmannur village of Pallakkad district of Kerala during their fieldwork of 2016. The village is situated in the relatively remote part of Mannarkad forest reserve in the state of Kerala. Chemmannur village has three hamlets located within its boundaries. They are Chemmannur, Seenkara, and Oosatihiyoor hamlets, and all the three are part of the Irula tribe. The total population of the Chemmannur village is 1153 of which 558 are male and 595 are females as per the ICDS data. Gender discrimination is not that prevalent in the village; the Panchayat president (ST category) and ward member (general category) are female candidates, and 52.2% of the total attendees in the previous Gram Sabha were also women and they have a significant role in the decision-making process. The total number of households in the Chemmannur village is 304, out of which 53.9% are pucca houses, 31.9% are semi-pucca houses, and 14.1% are kaccha houses. There has been large-scale migration to this region from 1950s from various parts of Kerala and Tamil Nadu. Attappady was an untapped and resource-rich area which made it suitable for cultivation, and also the abundance of valuable forest resource attracted settlers to the region. The village has three Anganwadis and a primary school which is government aided. There has been a steady increase in the number of the students who are enrolled in the school which is a positive indication of human development.

Chemmannur village belongs to Agali Gram Panchayat in Palakkad district of Kerala. Constant efforts made by the Village Panchayat and the Integrated Tribal Development Project (ITDP) in providing houses with toilets and toilets to those in need also helped in increasing the Open Defecation Free (ODF) numbers to 99%. This is a collective effort by the government and the people of the village to remove open defecation.

Initially toilets were built out of bamboo, bricks, and mud instead of cement under SBM. These works were mostly outsourced to contractors who implemented them very poorly. For example, in Sambarkode village initially common toilets were built and that too with bamboo, brick, and mud. After constant protest by the people only, it was changed to being built under individual households. After the baseline survey was carried out in late 2015, 52 target households were identified. About 52 toilets were built in the span of 15 months. Prior to the construction of toilets, both the male and female members of households had to attend Suchitwa Mission classes at ITDP. They were given instructions regarding specifications on building the toilet. Toilets that need to be constructed are of a double soak pit with a roof (RC, asbestos, or metallic sheet) and a fixed door. Piped water connection is not mandatory. It is up to the interest of people based on accessibility to water they build water tanks and install water taps. In some cases, people construct bathroom adjacent to the toilet or inside the toilet itself. Most of the toilets that were constructed were not attached to the households. During the starting of the construction Rs. 5000 was given as an aid for procurement of raw materials. The remaining was given in four instalments of which three instalments were issued upon producing the pictures of construction as directed during the classes. The final instalment will be issued only after the inspection by the Village Extension Officer (VEO) from the ITDP. The supervisor in each ward ensures that work progresses as per specification.

The toilets built under SBM and in general don't have proper water connection because of which they face huge difficulty in transporting water from public tap/ wells to their respective toilets (as terrain is mostly hilly). Under SBM people build toilets as per their wish. Some have separate bathing areas and washing areas. They keep a fixed door made of fibre or metal. In some cases, people spend money from their hand and build a bath area next to that. Some toilets in the hamlets built under SBM have been paved with tiles.

The SBM activity started in villages in late 2015 with baseline survey and construction of toilets started in 2016. Out of the total households surveyed 63% of them have heard or read about or seen something about the SBM; the rest that is 37% of the households were unaware of SBM. Majority of the households have known about SBM in the time frame of the last 12–24 months and the rest are aware about SBM in the last 12 months. Almost the same number of households is not aware of SBM; this shows that more efforts are required at ground level. People came to know about SBM from the beginning of 2016. The main source of awareness about SBM for the majority of households was from village-level meetings by NGO, Attappady Social Service Organization (ASSO), and Kudumbashree self-help groups meetings. ASSO gave classes on capacity building and on sanitation practices while they were implementing their projects in tribal hamlets. Almost the same number of households had come to know about SBM through newspapers. Radio and wall paintings have contributed least towards the awareness about SBM among people.

After the implementation of the AHADS project in villages, tribal houses got toilets. The toilets made by AHADS and influx of settlers into the region have given tribal people a notion about the importance of safe defecation and the importance of toilets. Settlers constructed toilets between 1980 and 1990, whereas for tribes it's still in process. The toilets in village were constructed either by Gram Panchayat under various schemes like (SBM, TSC, various housing projects) or by the households using their own resources. The beneficiaries of government schemes were mostly BPL households which include ST, SC, and some OBC. Majority of the settlers constructed toilets on their own.

Most of the households have toilets with single soak pits. Settlers build single pits for toilets to save cost. In the hilly terrain, it's more economical. Depending on the income status of the households the size of the pit varies. The houses of settlers constructed recently have septic tanks. The AHADS houses constructed for tribal hamlets also have single pits. Toilets built under SBM have double soak pits. In tribal hamlets, the pits are close by as most of the houses are in close proximity. In the long run, close soak pits can lead to contamination of groundwater. Of the total number of households having toilets 82.76% have toilets without flush and the rest have flush. Households having toilets with flush are mostly from the upper income level and are of settlers. Households in which toilets have been constructed under SBM don't have toilets with flush.

Most of the toilets of the settlers have piped water connection either from their own well or Jalanidhi project of NABARD. They have separate storage tanks for water. But in tribal hamlet toilets do not have taps. The main reason for unavailability is the hilly terrain. Osathiyoor hamlet has acute water shortage issues. As a result, people depend on Panchayat distributed water. Only very few households of upper-class tribes have a hand wash facility inside the toilets, and they use liquid hand wash for cleaning the hands. Majority of the people in the village use a common wash area or another wash area adjacent to the toilet. The hand wash facility is related to the income of households. Of all the surveyed households only two toilets do not have any roof; this was mainly because the roof was temporarily made of organic material of coconut tree leaves and got damaged in the last rain. The majority of toilets of rich households have attached toilets (i.e. inside the house). For the toilets built under SBM having a roof is mandatory. The material used for the roof varies from concrete to aluminium sheets. However, most people prefer asbestos roof. As high as 90% of the households have fixed doors in their toilets, 3% of households do not have a door, 6% of households have a temporary door, and 1% of them have curtains. The toilets that use curtains are those of tribes who stay in the remote area of Chemmannur hamlet. In earlier times, households used door made of coconut tree leaves. The toilets of tribes which were constructed before 2005 used temporary doors. These doors would get damaged due to use. There are few households that have unfixed doors. Most of the toilets in the village are not attached to houses. As per Vastu Shastra, the toilets and bathrooms in a home must be separate and not attached, and the tribe also believes in having toilets separate from households. Building facility for differently abled is not that prominent in the village. About 39% of the household clean toilets more than once a week which shows that people have a habit of maintaining clean toilets. About 24% of the households are cleaning daily, and 14% are cleaning once in a week and once in a fortnight. Only 2% of the 150 households surveyed clean their toilets only once in a month; this is because they do not have access to cleaning material because of low income. About 32% of households are using only water which shows that people are not having access to better cleaning materials because of low income. About 47% of the households are using branded toilet cleaner for cleaning toilets which is due to awareness about using safe cleaning materials for cleaning toilets. The factors that motivated people to construct toilet in the last three years were the influence from government, family, and the NGO. Only a few people had constructed toilets as their houses were undergoing renovation.

Even though entire Attappady is declared as ODF, we identified four households during our survey which were not having toilets. Out of the four, three had toilets but it was completely damaged and not in state to be used; the remaining one house was a kaccha house made of silpaulin sheet and it hasn't constructed a toilet yet. Hence people of all the four households were dependent on the neighbour's toilet for defecating purposes and the people understood its importance and permitted the neighbours to use their toilet. This shows us that an HH not having a toilet doesn't mean that people are defecating in the open. Attempts are being made by the Grama Panchayat to construct toilets for the pending ones. The neighbour's house was in close vicinity and in three cases the neighbours were their relatives. The households were not willing to renovate the damaged toilet because they started using it as additional space to store their goods. During the PRA interaction, we understood the factors that hindered tribal people from not using toilets. They were social stigma, comfort in the open, and lack of adequate water.

Meet Sharma in 2017 spent his fieldwork period in Devarapalli village of Krishna district in Andhra Pradesh. Devarapalli is a comparatively large village hosting a population of 2710 as per the 2011 census constituting about 720 households. The village consists of people from mainly four different caste categories, namely GEN, BC, SC, and ST. The GEN category is dominated by the Reddy community, gauds dominate the OBC category, while madhiga and lampadi caste dominate among the SC and ST categories, respectively. The basis for domination is preliminary based on the occupation. The village presents heterogeneity with the presence of people from the broad caste categories of GEN, BC, SC, and ST.

Though the village doesn't have any penetration of SBM, it is nearing ODF with households (HHs) from every community aware about the importance of toilets and their maintenance. The toilets coverage in the village accounts to 83.33%. Also unobtrusive observations show that all of the family members having toilets in the households are using them for all the sanitation-related activities.

Even though Swachh Bharat Abhiyan is recently inducted in the Krishna district of Andhra Pradesh, it is exceptional to find that 42 respondents out of sample size of 50 are aware about the Swachh Bharat Abhiyan. Most of the respondents came to know about SBM with the help of television. People are preferring to read newspapers like 'Sakshi' and 'Eenadu'. Apart from these two mediums, SHGs in the village also contribute to the awareness but at a very low scale. A small portion of the respondents mentioned about the posters. Though posters about schemes like Sarva Siksha Abhiyan and Beti Padhao Beti Bachao were found in the village, posters regarding SBM were not found. People's perception about the toilets and their usage can be used to show their awareness about the intention of the programme. With the HHs survey, it came out that more than 90% of respondents believe that their struggle has gone down with usage of toilets as compared to open defecation. This shows that people are aware about the benefits of having and using toilets. About 86% of respondents believe that women in family can ensure their privacy because of toilets.

The Swachh Andhra Mission was recently inducted in the Andhra state on 2 October 2017. It is quite surprising to see the toilet coverage in the village before SBM. This can be attributed to the overall health and sanitation awareness among villagers as out of the 46 HHs encountered with toilets, 69% are constructed by self-efforts. The data from the village revenue office states that presently approx. 83% of the HHs in the village are having toilets and 42 of the total HHs surveyed (50) had constructed toilets before SBM. Several unobtrusive observations and household visits over a period of one and half months in the Devarapalli village can conclude that the villagers having toilets at home and using them are mostly using branded liquid toilet cleaners like 'Domex' or 'Harpic'. It also came out during analysis that only 4% of the HHs surveyed were cleaning toilets once in a fortnight. Here's some statistics related to toilet maintenance practices in Devarapalli. All the HHs surveyed had a septic tank type of toilet. Also, more than 90% of the HHs surveyed had their toilets located in the backyard or front of the house. About 78% of respondents believe that overflow, bad smell, and mosquitoes are the result of poorly maintained toilets.

Out of the 50 HHs surveyed, 6 HHs could be found that did not have toilets at their home and had to defecate in open areas. A conversation with them gave an idea about several issues because of which they do not have toilets at home. The findings suggest that the HHs devoid of toilets can be attributed to some structural and planning issues on part of the government. Most households could remember Gandhi's specs logo and relate it to SBM and linked SBM with PM Modi. It was observed that most villagers were aware about cleaning activities carried under SBM. Though very few related SBM with toilet maintenance and its sustainable usage, household (HH) actions were reflective of the emphasis given to the maintenance of toilets. Most HHs cleaned toilets more than twice a week and they were using toilet's specific liquid cleaners. The toilet construction efforts show that 22% of the toilets constructed were because of the mixed efforts of the government and HHs. Because construction of toilets started way before SBM, attitudinal changes have taken place over the years which reflect in the high number of toilet users among the HHs.

From the data available via the Gram Panchayat and the VRO office, 16% of the HHs are still engaged in the open defecation and it was visible during transect walks in the Harijanwada area and field visits. The reasons coming out of the HH survey practicing open defecation were more of structural issues pertaining to the government rather than HHs not willing to construct toilets.

The overall well-being, present health status of the families in the village, and its comparison with the Krishna district and state health status can be attributed to the villagers' importance given to the health and allied activities. One contradicting viewpoint is people's perception towards correlating respect with ownership of the toilets. It shows that villagers' perceptions can still be improved in terms of the psychological importance given to toilet ownership. The IEC has been effective in dissemination of the message of sanitation; a substantial share of the budget is given to the advertisement and allied ways to reach people. However, it is doubtful whether such knowledge will translate to behaviour change.

Rohit, Sneh, and Vyom spent about eight weeks of the autumn of 2017 in the village Billi Markundi in Sonbhadra district of Uttar Pradesh. The village has 3761 households with a total population of 21082 (2011 census), of which 11080 are men and 10002 are women. All the above households are divided into Above Poverty Line (2905 HHs) and Below Poverty Line (856 HHs) categories on the basis of household income. However, the present footfall is around 60000. According to Village Panchayat, the population also reaches near 1 lakh during peak mining season. Billi Markundi village is divided into 15 wards and 9 hamlets (tolas). According to our household survey, 28% of houses are pucca houses, 51% of houses are semi-pucca houses, while the remaining 21% are kuccha houses. Those houses which are near to power plants and cement factories are occupied by retired officers and working employees and are generally pucca houses. These types of houses are homogeneously mixed in the village; however, semi-pucca houses were more prominent than kuccha and pucca houses. Out of 3761 HHs in the village, 2905 HHs fall under APL category and 856 HHs fall under BPL category. Billi Markundi has 2361 families falling under OBC category followed by SC, General, and ST category HHs. The literacy rate of Billi Markundi village is 62.53% in which male literacy rate is 72.91% whereas female literacy rate is 54.16%. The literacy rate for females is better than that of those in Sonbhadra district as well as Uttar Pradesh state. Male literacy rate in the village is worse in comparison to district- and state-level figures.

They surveyed about 150 HHs. That out of 74 pucca houses in the village there were 12 houses which did not have toilets. The main reasons being, first, they were recently built and the family did not have money to invest in toilets. Second, the family used the neighbours' toilet. Similarly, out of 52 semi-pucca houses, only 17 had toilets, and out of 24 kuccha houses only 4 had toilets. The mere 32.7% toilet coverage in semi-pucca houses and 16.67% toilet coverage in kuccha houses give us the target to put our resources into. The target respondents were divided in four categories as R1, R2, R3, and R4 based on the SEC category of these respondents. The responses were recorded on the basis of strata such that 20% of respondents are from each R1 and R2 categories. And there are 30% respondents from R3 and R4 categories. These strata are defined from the type of house and literacy status. They were considered to keep diversity in our sample and to get a holistic perspective. The survey results suggested that about 87% of the respondents were aware about SBM or at least had read/heard/seen about SBM at some point of time which indicates that SBM has a good wide spread in the village and a significant number of people are aware of the government programme. But the people going for open defecation do not really wish to take action by themselves even after such widespread awareness and local government fully operational in this arena.

The Swachh Bharat Abhiyaan started in 2014, i.e., about 36 months back. The results make us believe that when the Swachh Bharat Abhiyaan was announced there was a lot of hoax around it, but in recent times this has come down as only

8% of the respondents said that they have heard about SBM in the last six months. About 42% respondents said that they last heard about SBM about 12–24 months back, and 27% respondents said that they last heard about SBM about 24–36 months back, i.e., at the time of introduction or announcement of Swachh Bharat Abhiyaan. The toilets constructed in the village were mainly of the double soak pit type which is in accordance with the scheme of SBM as it also requires beneficiaries to build a double soak pit. About 54% of the toilets had a double soak pit construction. About 21% of the toilets had a septic tank. About 25% of the toilets had a single soak pit construction.

Everyone in the family is using the toilets and there are no social barriers among the members of the family. There is no discrimination against women or children to not use toilets. In fact it is observed that villagers are concerned about safety and privacy of the women and hence they have constructed toilets. Analytically 2% preferred that only women should go to the toilets, and 3% believed that only men and women should use the toilets. The main motivation behind building toilets is found to be ‘to avoid inconveniences caused during rainy season’. Sonbhadra is a district well known for snakes, and it is thus dangerous to go out in the open for defecation during monsoon. The next most important motivation is ‘safety and privacy of women’. The women are looked at with a lot of respect, and hence their privacy is an important motivating factor to build toilets inside the house. The social pressure in recent times has actually elevated the rate at which the toilets are being constructed. Whereas respondents have shown disagreement with factors like marriage in family or persuasion by leaders to construct toilets as the reasons to construct toilets.

The HHs with no toilets were asked reasons for not having toilets. The major reason was lack of sufficient money to build the toilet. Owing to low wages of the villagers this seems a justified explanation. The next important factor that causes hindrance is that there were more important things at their disposal whenever they had access to money. The villagers are used to saving money in order to construct the toilet but most of the time their savings were being used up for some other emergency work. The most disturbing factor is that ‘It doesn’t matter we have toilet or not’. This shows that villagers are well aware of the need and merits of having a toilet. Also it tells us that villagers actually wish to have a toilet and they are not able to construct under compulsion. The other factor is ‘We don’t like men and women going to the same toilet’ but with the responses it has become clear that there is no social constraint or psychological constraint in the mind so as not to use the same toilet with the opposite gender.

In 2017 Rohit and Sakshi did their fieldwork in two villages (Cheekhla and Khunadari) in Udaipur district of Rajasthan. Cheekhla and Khunadari villages are located in Kotra block and Kherwada block, respectively. Cheekhla had a total population of 8142 people. There were about 1352 houses in Cheekhla while Khunadari had a total population of 611 people with 133 houses. Cheekhla is a tribal-dominated village, while Khunadari is a non-tribal village with a substantial number of people from Brahmins, Bhils, Rajputs, etc. In the survey it was found that the people in both the villages thought that toilets have certain advantages over open defecation and it is needed particularly for women in terms of providing safety. Most benefitted by constructing toilets and saw them as a useful resource. People in Cheekhla didn't consider maintaining toilets as difficult and agreed that toilets were changing their lives.

In Khunadari, people acknowledge the fact that privacy for women, respect in society, safety, and self-esteem go up with construction of toilets but think that toilets lead to an increase in workload or increase in water consumption and contamination of ground water. In Khunadari, 66% of the surveyed households had a toilet. Out of these 66%, in 64% of the houses the toilet is used by everyone in the family. About 34% of the surveyed households did not have access to toilets and were either using public toilets or resorting to open defecation. In Cheekhla, 72% of the surveyed people have toilets but only 16% use toilets selectively or do not use them at all. In Khunadari, majority, 51% of the households, were self-constructed, without any help. About 14% of people built their toilets with help from government/NGOs. Only 5% are built under SBM. In Cheekhla, 40% of the toilets were built under SBM and 32% by NGO – Seva Mandir. All the toilets constructed in both the villages were funded by the government. It was found that local-level leaders played a pivotal role in getting the toilets; the NGOs and the community-based organisations were involved in the construction of toilets. There were certain pull factors such as the toilets provided convenience specifically for elderly and women of the household. In some cases the households became ready to construct the toilet because the children were getting married. In many cases children pressurised the parents to construct the toilet.

However, this was not without the attendant problems. Most families were still defecating in the open. The major demotivating factors were: not having space to build toilet, lack of money, water shortage, one toilet not enough for all family members, there are more important things than toilet, toilet degrades quality of water, won't like men and women use the same toilet, and the fear of the pit filling up. The quality of toilets constructed under SBM in both villages is quite different. In Cheekhla, toilets have a permanent roof and door whereas in Khunadari, toilets constructed under SBM have temporary roofs and proper water facility is also not available in these toilets. Toilet constructed by Seva mandir is Ecosan, i.e., ash is used instead of water. The degraded waste is then used in the agricultural fields as organic manure.

Tushar Badheria did his fieldwork in 2017 at the Girirajpura and Amli villages of Tonk district in Rajasthan. Girirajpura village is situated on the land given by the Forest Department for rehabilitation of villagers who used to stay inside the core area of Ranthambore National Tiger Reserve and is located just five kilometres from the forest area. The village comprises people rehabilitated from two villages – Mordungri and Padra which used to be inside the Ranthambore Tiger Reserve and were rehabilitated by the government. Total land area of the village was 100 acres and out of which 90 acres were agricultural land. The total population of the village is 216 with 51 households in 27 houses. Literacy rate of the village is very low as there was no government or private institution for education in the forest area and the nearest school was 10–12 km away, so most of the adults in the village are illiterate; only six people in the village are graduates. But after rehabilitating to Girirajpura all children started schooling, as it was provided by an NGO free of cost and school was in the village only. Sex ratio of the village is 110 males per 100 females. Literacy rate of the village is around 24%. Only four households are BPL households in the village. The village consists of only Gurjar caste of the Hindu religion and is of OBC class. The people in the village were rehabilitated from two different villages named Mordungri and Padra, and hence they live in two hamlets and the hamlets are named on the names of their old villages. Both the groups in the hamlets follow their cultures and celebrate all the festivals that are celebrated by Hindus.

Major occupation of the villagers in the forest was cattle rearing, and they used to sell milk in the city. But after rehabilitation, cattle were not able to produce as much milk as they used to in the forest due to less fodder availability as the village has less water availability. Hence now the major occupation of the villagers is farming and they grow crops like urad, bajra, peanuts, mustard, wheat, etc. They also have some cattle and sell the milk in Sawai Madhopur City. Aside from this, villagers are cooperative in their farming works as most of the tube wells are dry and they share water for irrigation facilities.

The Gram Panchayat had stopped the ration from the public distribution centre of the villagers who were not opting for toilets in their respective houses. In village the Girirajpura Panchayat has done the same and gave warning to the Girirajpura villagers that if they have not built toilets by 31 March 2018, their ration supply will be stopped. To spread awareness of SBM, Uday Learning Centre (NGO) has also started explaining to people about the benefits of building toilets. The Panchayat forced the villagers of Amli to build toilets in their houses, which was successful as 75% of the houses in Amli now have toilets. But some of the villagers keep their toilets locked and use them only in emergencies like the rainy season or at night. So to increase the usage of toilets, the Panchayat office has come up with a new movement against people who are going for open defecation. Also from the figure we can see that villagers in Amli have built two toilets in their houses to get Rs. 24000 (Rs. 12000 for each). After the Panchayat office inspects the toilet, it writes the name of the person who owns the house and writes the amount of money given to the household. Through this method Panchayat members spread awareness of SBM by writing the details on the toilet gate so that more and more people will build toilets.

In village Girirajpura none of the households have toilets in their houses. Gramin Shiksha Kendra, also called Uday Learning School, has a primary school in village Girirajpura which has built toilets for both boy and girl students. As the toilet is built in the school area by this NGO is trying to implant a habit in children of using toilets rather than going for OD. By this habit, it is trying to remove the old habit of OD from the young generations. In village Amli 75% of households are having toilets in their homes and to increase the usage level of these toilets a whistle-blow drive is being carried out by the Panchayat office, and it's been ordered by the collector to make village open defecation free by 31 March 2018. The collector had sent letters to the villagers to stop practice of open defecation in the villages, which were pasted at the prominent places. It also informed the villagers that those who have built their toilets in their house should attach the papers of toilets with bank passbook, Adhar card, and Bhamashah card in order to get the benefits of government schemes, and those who fail to do so will not get free ration through the ration shops.

Village Amli is having 75% households with toilets in their houses and there were several reasons for them to build toilets in their houses. Most people were forced by the leaders to build the toilet, and also some people in the village built toilets for the safety of women. Due to improvement in education level children are also forcing their parents to build toilets for health and hygiene. Villagers used to follow each other; if one person is building a toilet in his house then others will also start building toilets. Villagers have now started building toilets in their houses when they are renovating or building their house as this will not cost much to them in comparison to building a toilet alone.

In village Girirajpura there was no toilet because the main constraint was the money; people were not having enough salary and also they have been rehabilitated from the forest, so to change the habit of OD is quite tough for them as it will change their behaviour aspects. Poverty is the main reason for not a building toilet in the house. The residents believed that toilet construction at home is a waste of money and time as the area suffers from acute water shortages, so having a toilet will increase water consumption by 5–10 litres per person per day. So villagers believe that building a toilet and maintaining it is a difficult task as it will increase the workload of women as they will be carrying water from the water source to the households because none of the households are having water connections also.

Sachin Arya conducted his fieldwork in the village Saree Peepli in Pratapgarh district of Rajasthan. Saree Peepli is situated on the boundary of Sitamata Wildlife Sanctuary, partly situated inside the boundary and partly situated outside. The village is spread across forest, and low-height hills of Aravalli cross the villages at places. Surrounded by the lush green forests and teak trees, river Jakham enhances the beauty of the village that flows through it and divides the village in half. Saree Peepli is a small village of around 43 in the 2011 census (actual households are ~90). The houses are spread on both the sides of the road and some houses inside the fields. Densely populated area in the village is approximately one kilometre towards both sides of the road. The population density is quite low. The population of the village was 224 as per the census and out of which 113 were male and 111 were female. Literacy rate is extremely low at 37.5% due to mainly poverty and reluctance towards getting their wards educated. Only five to six households have toilets in the village. Open defecation is prevalent but still villagers are inclined towards building the toilets due to the problems they face of insect bites and wild animal attack in the forest, but the major problem is the funds; many toilets we saw in the village were half build and because those people didn't receive the funds promised under SBM, they didn't build the toilets further. To encourage people to build toilets, a practice has been adopted to write 'Pyara Ghar' on the houses that have toilets and mark the houses without toilets with an 'X'. This is almost equivalent to public shaming, and residents feel embarrassed if an 'X' is painted on their door.

In the survey about 58% of the respondents reported that they did not know about the Swachh Bharat Abhiyan. To 'motivate' people to construct toilets in this village also, the Panchayat stopped providing ration through PDS if the households did not agree to build the toilets. Secondly, the Gram Panchayat started a campaign of 'Pyara Ghar'; they would write 'Paya Ghar' on the front walls of the houses which have constructed toilets and would put a cross (X) mark at the front of the houses without toilets in white paint. In a controversial case, the collector of the nearby district of Pratapgarh had issued an order for the teachers and other people of the village to click photos and record videos of people taking a dump in the open and soon the photos and videos were uploaded on the internet. It was alleged that one lady took her life due to this. After this, the practice stopped.

In the village of Saree Peepli, only 37.5% of houses are having toilets. Most of the people built these toilets under SBM, and people who have used their money are waiting for the reimbursement of the money by the government. Many of the toilets in households were stopped midway during the construction as the people did not get the amount promised under SBM, so the toilets constructed are lacking basic facilities such as inside tap water, flush, wash basin, etc. In simple terms, they are just a structure with a pit and toilet seat. Village Saree Peepli was not having toilets in their households, and there were several reasons for them to build toilets in their houses. The reasons for construction of toilets that we came across while enquiring with the villagers were the convenience of the family members and the privacy of the woman members of the family. As the village was on the boundary of a wildlife sanctuary and a few villages of the Gram Panchayat fall inside the boundary of Sitamata Wildlife Sanctuary, the risk of animal attack and insect bite is also high. Many times, the villagers see panthers and other wild animals when going out in the morning for open defecation. The funds promised under SBM worked as a catalyst in the construction of the toilets, and people were motivated to construct the toilets as the amount they invested in the toilets was reimbursed by the government to the extent of Rs. 12000.

Notes

1 This section has extracts from the unpublished PhD dissertation of the second author.

2 Article 243-G of the Constitution of India provides that the states/ UTs may, by law, endow the Panchayats with such powers and authority as may be necessary to enable them to function as institutions of self-government and to prepare plans for economic development and social justice and their implementation including those in relation to the matters listed in the Eleventh Schedule (GOI, 2001).

4 Survey of Three States

Background to the Survey

Sanitation behaviour depends on the economic, social, and infrastructural environment (De, 2018). An in-depth understanding of sanitation behaviour is possible through a survey of households. We have attempted to conduct such analysis based on quantitative and qualitative data. In this study, we have considered the households' economic, social, and infrastructural backdrop. We have selected households from varied socio-economic backgrounds to generate a representative sample. To make it representative of the country, we have covered states from different regions and sociocultural backdrops. For the quantitative analysis, multiple stratified random sampling methods were applied to select households. The study was carried out in Telangana, Bihar, and Rajasthan. The following observations were made on state-wise policy implications.

Telangana

Telangana has the highest number of ODF villages. To provide comprehensive sanitation in the state, Telangana has secured the first position with the highest number of ODF villages in the country in implementing the Swachh Bharat Mission Phase-II programme; about 13737 villages out of 14200 (96.74%) were positioned in the ODF plus list. As per the dashboard of NITI Aayog for 2020–1, Telangana was ranked second in the country in providing clean water and sanitation. To achieve this milestone and sustain sanitation activities, the state has implemented a wide variety of sanitation activities like the construction of public toilets, community toilets, mobile toilets, and She toilets (meant exclusively for women) in 142 towns.

Telangana is the first state in India to initiate gender integration in sanitation. It involved the Self Help Group (SHG) members in acting as sanitation messengers in the community to promote safe hygiene practices by toilet users in the community and entrusted model contracts and offered Rs 2500 per toilet for operations and maintenance of toilets in urban areas. At present, 170 such contracts have been assigned to SHG entrepreneurs. Telangana adopted the state-owned Faecal Sludge and Septage Management (FSSM) policy on 29 September 2018. To address the state's sanitation issues and effective implementation of the

DOI: 10.4324/9781032726267-4

FSSM policy, the government has explored the integrated approach by developing the institutional framework and action plans to sustain the implementation of the FSSM policy.

Bihar

Bihar is one of the most highly populated states in the country; as per NITI Ayog's Poverty Index Report for 2021, over 50% of the population in Bihar belongs to multidimensional poverty. According to the press release by the State Public Health Engineering Department, the groundwater has been contaminated with toxic substances, i.e., fluoride, arsenic, and iron. Eleven districts had fluoride contamination, 14 districts had arsenic poisoning, and 12 districts had excessive iron content. In these circumstances, the state government initiated the Chief Minister's Rural Drinking Water Scheme (Har Ghar Nal ka Jal) in 2016 to provide piped drinking water, free from water contamination and within permissible limits of fluoride, arsenic, and iron

Health and Sanitation. As per the fourth edition of NITI Ayog on Health Index for 2019–20, Bihar was ranked second poorest performer with an index score of 31 and placed in the least improved category among the larger states in India. The Government of Bihar has been implementing various health programmes and infrastructure like hospitals, medical colleges, emergency services, labs and pharmacies, etc. and has become a medical hub. The Health Department of Bihar is functioning as a coalition with the State Health Society and Bihar Medical Services and Infrastructure Corporation Limited (BMSICL), and at the grassroots level, health bodies are contributing to providing quality services.

According to the National Family Health Survey (NHFS-5), the toilet facility is available for 62% of households in Bihar, and the improved sanitation facility is accessible for 49.4%. As per the National Green Tribunal (NGT) study, more than 4000 deaths occurred due to air pollution-caused diseases.

Gujarat

Gujarat is one of the highly urbanised states with 42.60% of the urban population and an annual growth rate of 1.44%. Gujarat has been declared as the sixth ODF state in India. The Government of Gujarat developed the Water and Sanitation Management Organization (WASMO) in 2002 to engage the community in managing their water bodies and sanitation. Gujarat is one of the water crisis-facing states in the country. To provide safe drinking water and sewerage and sewage disposal services to the state population, the Gujarat Water Supply and Sewerage Board was formed and functioning under the GWSSB Act No. 18 of 1979. In line with the Jal Jeevan Mission (JJM), Gujarat has provided safe and sufficient drinking water through individual tap water connections for 68.63 lakhs of households (HHs) out of 93.03 lakhs of HHs in rural Gujarat. The state enacted the state policy for Faecal Sludge and Septage Management (FSSM) in 2017 to achieve sustainable and safe sanitation in 31 cities of Gujarat.

Sanitation Intervention: A Multifaceted Intervention

Sanitation is a multifaceted intervention having inclusive management of water, drainage, waste management, etc., to intervene on a large scale. In India, the sanitation coverage was less than 1% in 1947. After independence, the central government has been implementing various sanitation schemes, viz. the Central Rural Sanitation Program (1986), the Total Sanitation Campaign (1999), the Nirmal Bharat Abhiyan (2012) and the Swachh Bharat Abhiyan (2014), to achieve universal sanitation coverage. The Economic Survey (2020–1) recommended strengthening the sanitation and drinking water system to reduce India's infectious diseases and mortality rates. As per NFHS-5, it is observed that the utilisation rate of sanitation facilities has increased from 49% during 2015–16 to 70% during 2019–21. Rural sanitation increased from 37% to 65%, and urban sanitation has progressed from 70% to 82%. More than 70% of the population belonging to 411 districts across 707 districts got access to an improved source of sanitation. In some states, i.e., Odisha, Bihar, Jharkhand, and Ladakh, access to improved sanitation is limited to only 42–60% of the population. During the last 70 years, India has shown considerable development in improving access to safe drinking water. The government has introduced various schemes; according to the data released by NFHS-5, the urban areas have better access to safe drinking water than rural areas, and overall access to drinking water is more significant than before 2015–16 in 22 states.

The study settings are decided based on coverage and regional location. The first criteria would capture variation in the progress of sanitation coverage, and the second would capture the sociocultural variation. Accordingly, we have selected three states: Bihar, Telangana, and Gujarat. In 2017, Bihar had the lowest access at 30%, Telangana had medium access at 61%, and Gujarat had the highest access at 85%. According to the Ministry of Culture, Government of India, Bihar is in the North Central Culture Zone, Gujarat is in the West Culture Zone, and Telangana is in the South Culture Zone. Thus, these three states represent different cultures and cultural norms of India.[1] Bihar is in the Indo-Gangetic plain, Gujarat has semi-arid alluvial plains, and Telangana is located on the Deccan Plateau. Thus, these three regions are also different from geographical features having implications for access to water for sanitation. The depth of groundwater is lowest in Bihar (0.5–10 m below ground level) as compared to Telangana (0.63–69.5 m bgl) and Gujarat (5–61 m bgl). Figure 4.1 represents the sampling frame after the selection of states.

The Sampling Frame

We selected sample households for the study from the three states.[2] These samples were selected based on a multistage stratified random sampling approach. From each state, we selected the best-performing district (BPD) and the worst-performing district (WPD) based on the progress made in toilet coverage (Figure 4.2). We selected the best and the worst-performing blocks from each district, as blocks are the basic unit of planning and implementation in SBM. The best- and worst-performing Gram Panchayats (GPs) were selected from each block as GP is the

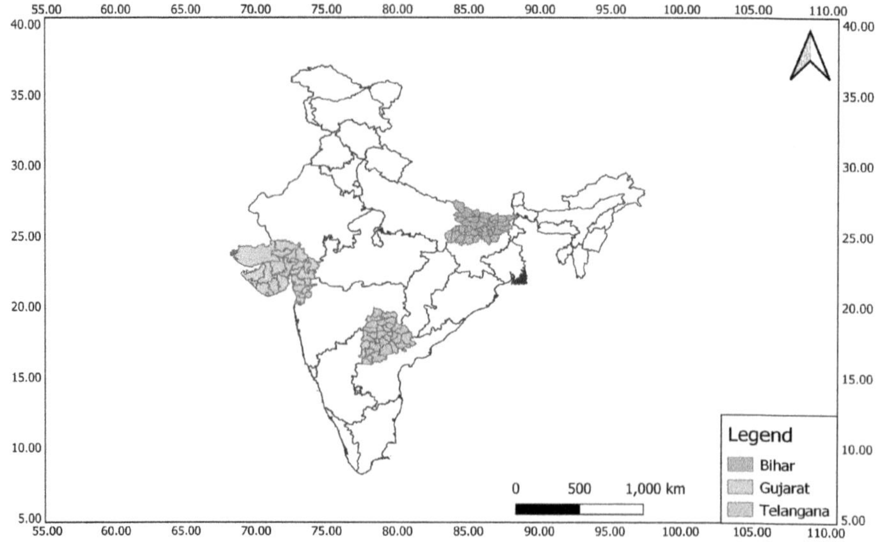

Figure 4.1 Sampling Frame after the Selection of States.

Source: Base map was taken from Wikimedia commons (https://commons.wikimedia.org/wiki/File:India-outline-map.jpg), modified by author

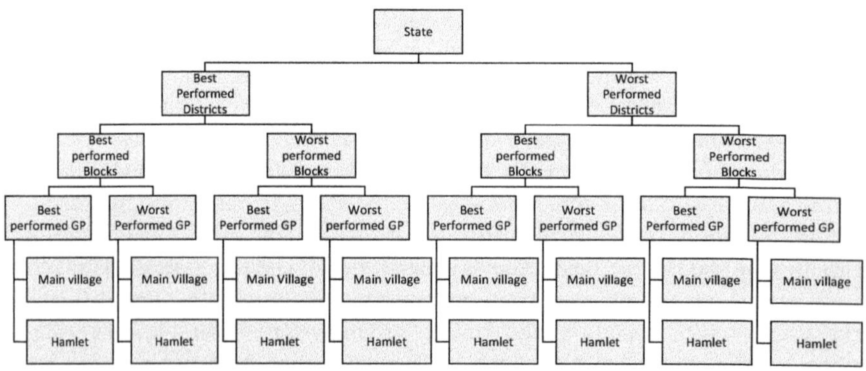

Figure 4.2 Sampling Frame after the Selection of States.

Source: Author's own creation

unit of collective behaviour change. Thus, from each state, we selected four Gram Panchayats.

Among the study states, Bihar lagged much behind Gujarat and Telangana for an extended period. According to the 2011 census, 67% of households had no toilet facility in rural India. The figure for Gujarat was 66% and for undivided Andhra Pradesh was 65% (Telangana separated from Andhra Pradesh in 2014). On the other hand, the percentage of rural households having no toilet was as high as 8% in Bihar. Similar scenarios emerge in urban India. While 13% of households did not have access to a toilet in urban India, the exact figure was much lower at 9% in Gujarat and 12% in undivided Andhra Pradesh. The percentage of urban households not having access to a toilet was again very high at 29% in Bihar.

Access to improved toilet facilities within premises was available to 25% of rural households in India in 2011. The same was higher in Gujarat and undivided Andhra Pradesh at 31% and 30%, respectively. However, the access to an improved toilet within premises was much lower at 14% in rural Bihar. Similarly, access to piped water facilities was available to 31% of rural households. Access to the same basic service was much higher in undivided Andhra Pradesh at 63% of households and in Gujarat at 56%. The access to the piped water supply was only 3% in rural Bihar.

In Gujarat, Sabarkantha and Dahod have been selected as the best- and worst-performing districts. Jhalod and Garbada blocks have been selected as the best- and worst-performing blocks from the Dahod district. Talod and Idar blocks have been selected as the best- and worst-performing blocks from the Sabarkantha district. Best-performing villages (Nalvai, Sarkari Raniyar, Salatpur, and Bhadreshar) and worst-performing villages (Dadur, Rupakheda, Vavdi, and Dungari) have been selected from the sample districts of Gujarat for the household survey (Figure 4.3). In Bihar, Sitamarhi and Samastipur districts have been selected as the best- and worst-performing districts. Parsouni and Runisaidpur were selected from the Sitamarhi district as the best- and worst-performing blocks. Sarairanjan and Hasanpur blocks have been selected from the Samastipur district as the best- and worst-performing blocks, respectively. The best-performing villages (Parsouni, Mahisar, Nargogi, and Marachi Ujagar) and the worst-performing villages (Gisara, Barheta, Musapur, and Rampur) have been selected from the sample districts of Bihar for the household survey (Figure 4.4).

Medak and Vikarabad districts from Telangana have been selected as the best- and worst-performing districts. Toparan and Chenguta have been selected from the Medak district as the best- and worst-performing blocks. Nawapet and Bashirabad blocks have been selected from the Vikarabad district as the

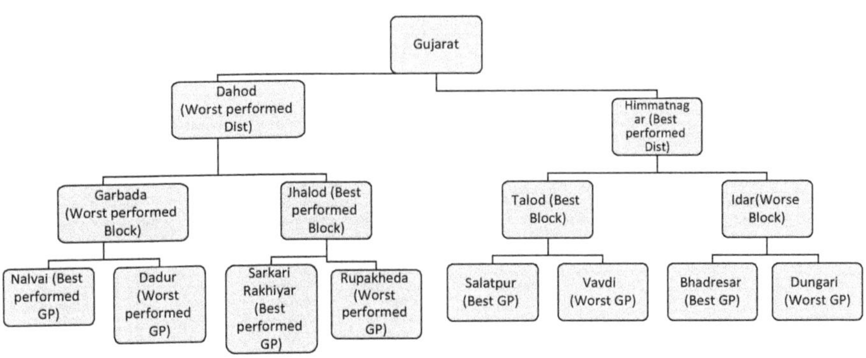

Figure 4.3 Sampling Plan for Gujarat.

Source: Author's own creation

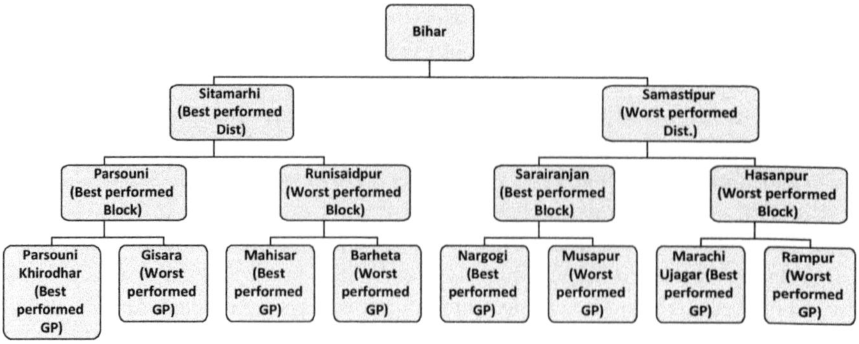

Figure 4.4 Sampling Plan for Bihar.

Source: Author's own creation

best- and worst-performing blocks. Best-performing villages (Malkapur, Ibrahimpur, Lingampally, and Allapur) and worst-performing villages (Konaipally, Wadiyaram, Madaram, and Neelapally) have been selected from the sample districts of Telangana for the household survey (Figure 4.5).

One of the best-performing villages was Malkapur in Medak district in Telangana. The total number of households in the village was 344. During the baseline survey of 2012, the village had already constructed 268 toilets, and the current status demonstrates 100% achievement in toilet construction in the village. In another best-performing village of the same district, out of 531 households, 520 constructed toilets during 2016–18. Neelapally, a worst-performing village in the same state, had 204 households with only 25 constructed toilets and 20 other toilets under construction at the survey. The rest of the households did not have access to a toilet.

We selected households through systematic random sampling from the main village of the GP and a hamlet close to the village. The process of random selection

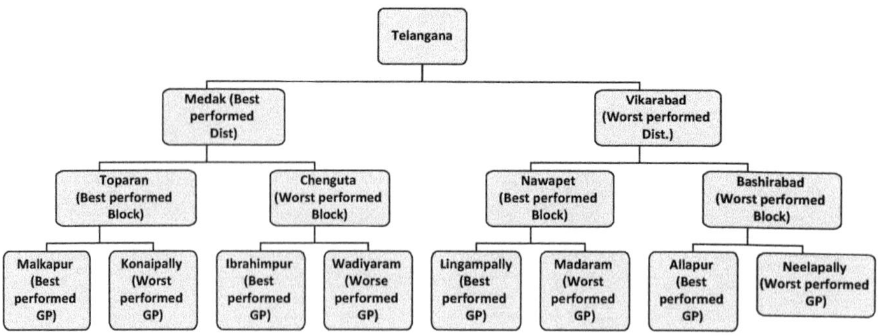

Figure 4.5 Sampling Plan for Telangana.

Source: Author's own creation

was done by first selecting a household (selected using random numbers) and then selecting every kth household (k is the ratio of population size to the desired sample size) from a village. This process was repeated in every village. Thus, the sample included every part of the village and every socio-economic stratum. Using a structured questionnaire, we collected quantitative data for the study from the household (HH) surveys. The study covered 1252 households across the three states. The details of the number of samples selected from different states, districts, blocks, and villages are given in Table 4.1. Pilot testing of the research has been done with 30 households each from the Sabarkantha and Samastipur districts of Gujarat and Bihar, respectively. The survey questionnaire included information on various social, physical, and behavioural indicators. The social, physical, and behavioural changes variables are gender, age, prestige/status, availability of water, cultural and social norms, awareness, intention, convenience, privacy, security, affordability, cleanliness, and attitude towards maintaining toilets and sustaining sanitation services. We assured all respondents that we would not share their personal information with anyone; the information would only be used for research purposes; we also briefed them about the importance of the research in positively impacting people around the country.

Qualitative Study

The qualitative analysis was done through in-depth study and structured and unstructured interviews of officials, masons, and political and social leaders. A focus group discussion (FGD) of households was also conducted for data collection. Participatory Rural Appraisal (PRA) was conducted to understand the household's perception of their social environment, social infrastructure, and resource availability. It was essential to understand the underlying factors that triggered the need for a toilet in people and the conditions that facilitated and motivated people to use toilets. Apart from in-depth interviews and FGDs, the study also used a relatively new technique in qualitative research design, which is very useful in studying consumer behaviour – this is the Zaltman Metaphor Elicitation Technique (Z-MET). The technique's uniqueness is its ability to bring up the issues from the users' perspective rather than being guided by the conception of the researchers.

Profile of Respondents

Among 1252 respondents of the primary survey, 69% were heads of households (HHs), while only 30% of the respondents were the other members of the HHs. More than 80% of the respondents were heads of households in Dahod. Medak had an almost equal share of responses from both members and the head of the HHs (Table 4.2). The gender composition of respondents and the head of households is also crucial for understanding sanitation behaviour because female members of the households are likely to receive higher benefits than men from sanitation due to enhanced privacy and convenience. There is a wide variation in the gender composition of the respondents. In Bihar, 61% of respondents were male, while in Gujarat, it was 83%. The percentage of male respondents was highest in Dahod at

Table 4.1 Distribution of Sample Across States, Districts, and Blocks

State	*Districts*	*Blocks*												*Total*
		Runnisaidpur	*Parsouni*	*Sarairanjan*	*Hasanpur*	*Idar*	*Talod*	*Jhalod*	*Gadbada*	*Toparan*	*Chenguta*	*Nawaped*	*Basheerabad*	
Bihar	Sitamarhi	101	128											229
	Samastipur			102	110									212
	Total	101	128	102	110									441
Gujarat	Sabarkantha					105	98							203
	Dahod							106	100					206
	Total					105	98	106	100					409
Telangana	Medak									101	100			201
	Vikarabad											50	151	201
	Total									101	100	50	151	402
Total		101	128	102	110	105	98	106	100	101	100	50	151	1252

Source: Own Primary Survey, 2018

Table 4.2 Average Number of Members at the Households

	Bihar			*Gujarat*			*Telangana*			*All*
Gender of Household Members	*Sitamarhi*	*Samastipur*	*Total*	*Sabarkantha*	*Dahod*	*Total*	*Medak*	*Vikarabad*	*Total*	
Male	3.83	3.28	3.56	2.46	3.16	2.81	2.43	2.87	2.65	3.02
Female	3.45	3.02	3.24	2.25	2.98	2.62	2.34	2.57	2.46	2.78
Total	7.28	6	7	5	6	5	5	5	5	6

Source: Own Primary Survey, 2018

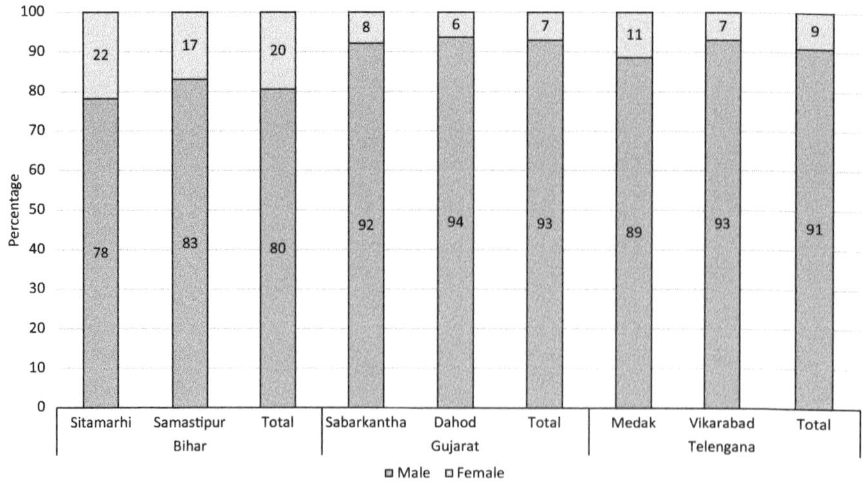

Figure 4.6 Household Head by Gender.

Source: Own Primary Survey

90%. Only 12% of the total households of three states reported women as head of the HHs (Table 4.2). In the sample, Bihar was reported to have the most female-headed households (Figure 4.6).

The number of members in the household also has implications for the construction of toilets. It may be challenging to construct a toilet in a large family due to the possibility of conflicting opinions on sanitation behaviour among family members. More members make it difficult to use the toilet during the same period. Furthermore, the number of female members in the household vis-à-vis number of male members also matters when deciding on toilet construction within the dwelling. In our sample, on average, there are six members per household, with a higher number of males than females. The household size is most prominent in Bihar compared to the other two states (Table 4.2). The age of the household head is also likely to have implications for sanitation behaviour. Younger people may be more open to behaviour changes in sanitation than the older people who may resist behaviour change due to entrenched social norms. But some may prefer toilet use due to their restricted mobility. We find that the heads are between 30 and 45 years in a substantial proportion of sample households. In an equally substantial proportion of sample households, the heads are 45–60 years old. Hence, it seems the sample households are young enough to decide in favour of using a toilet.

The education of the household members is vital to consider as it may have implications for the acceptability of modern progressive behaviour such as the use of toilets. We have enquired about the highest level of education of male and female members of the households. We observed that illiteracy is more common among females. In Bihar, more than half of the households have all female members illiterate. The highest level of education among males goes up to postgraduation or professional degree. But females' highest education is restricted to the 12th standard of schooling (Table 4.3). The disparity in education between males and females is highest in Bihar.

Socio-Economic Status of the Household

The social identity of the household may play an essential role in sanitation behaviour because social norms regarding sanitation may differ across social and religious groups. In our survey, 93% of households were Hindu (Table 4.4). Only 3% of households were Muslims, and 4% were Christians. Sample households from Bihar and Gujarat did not have any Christian households, while in Telangana, 11% of the households belonged to the Christian community. More than 90% of the sample households belonged to socially backward casts (Table 4.5). The representation of upper caste households in the sample was highest in Bihar. The distribution of castes varied widely across districts. While the Dahod district of Gujarat had 82% scheduled tribe (ST) households in the sample, the same is as low as around 3% in Samastipur in Bihar and Vikarabad in Telangana. Bihar had a higher share of the scheduled caste (SC) population than two other states. About 51% of the households belonged to other backward castes (OBC) in Telangana, which was higher than the other two states.

Occupation and Economic Status

The primary occupation of the household has implications for the personal attitudes of household members, especially the head of the household. The majority of the members of the households were engaged in their agricultural fields or employed as wage labour in others' fields. The employment scenario in Bihar was much different from Gujarat and Telangana. Only around a quarter of the households in Bihar were engaged in agriculture as a primary occupation, while the same for Gujarat and Telangana is more than three-fourth. Households engaged as regular wage earners were comparatively much higher in Bihar compared to Gujarat and Telangana. Exposure to households outside traditional occupations such as agriculture may have positive implications for toilet use.

Approximately 10% of the households worked as agricultural labour. Employment in agriculture is seasonal and highly uncertain. The percentage of households engaged in casual labour was much higher in Bihar than in Gujarat and Telangana. Around 3% of households were also engaged in casual labour, again highest in Bihar. Employment opportunity as casual labour is subject to uncertainty and low pay. With higher uncertainty in employment and lower wages, the group does not generate demand for sanitation. Stable employment such as government jobs is rarely available among members of the survey households. For example, among 1252 households surveyed, only one household in the Sitamarhi district had a government job (Table 4.6).

The primary occupation of households across villages in the same state varied widely. The most crucial primary occupation of the households in the best-performing villages was agriculture. In Malkapur village, the best-performing village

Table 4.3 Percentage Distribution of Households by Highest Level of Education of Household Members

	Bihar		*Gujarat*		*Telangana*		*All*	
	Male	*Female*	*Male*	*Female*	*Male*	*Female*	*Male*	*Female*
Illiterate	39.91	52.15	11	25.92	11.44	25.37	21.33	34.98
Till 10th standard	32.43	36.05	47.92	46.7	51	41.29	43.45	41.21
Till 12th standard	9.75	11.79	41.08	27.38	37.56	33.33	28.91	23.8
Graduation	8.16						2.88	
Postgraduation	1.13						0.4	
Professional degree	8.62						3.04	
Total	100	100	100	100	100	100	100	100

Source: Own Primary Survey, 2018

Table 4.4 Percentage Distribution of Households by Religion

Religion	*Bihar*			*Gujarat*			*Telangana*			*All*
	Sitamarhi	*Samastipur*	*Total*	*Sabarkantha*	*Dahod*	*Total*	*Medak*	*Vikarabad*	*Total*	
Hindu	91.70	98.11	94.78	98.03	100.00	99.02	87.56	82.59	85.07	93.05
Muslim	8.30	1.89	5.22	1.97	0.00	0.98	4.98	1.49	3.23	3.19
Christian	0.00	0.00	0.00	0.00	0.00	0.00	6.97	15.92	11.44	3.67
Jain	0.00	0.00	0.00	0.00	0.00	0.00	0.50	0.00	0.25	0.08
Total	100.00	100.00	100.00	100.00	100.00	100.00	100.00	100.00	100.00	100.00

Source: Primary Survey, 2018

Table 4.5 Percentage Distribution of Households by Castes

Caste	*Bihar*			*Gujarat*			*Telangana*			*All*
	Sitamarhi	*Samastipur*	*Total*	*Sabarkantha*	*Dahod*	*Total*	*Medak*	*Vikarabad*	*Total*	
ST	4.80	3.30	4.08	23.15	81.55	52.57	6.47	3.48	4.98	20.21
SC	40.61	55.66	47.85	38.92	18.45	28.61	34.33	37.81	36.07	37.78
OBC	36.24	34.43	35.37	37.93	0.00	18.83	49.25	52.74	51.00	34.98
General	18.34	6.60	12.70	0.00	0.00	0.00	9.95	5.97	7.96	7.03
Total	100.00	100.00	100.00	100.00	100.00	100.00	100.00	100.00	100.00	100.00

Source: Primary Survey, 2018
Legend: ST – scheduled tribe; SC – scheduled caste; OBC – other backward caste

Table 4.6 Percentage Distribution of Households by Primary Occupation

Primary Occupation	*Bihar*			*Gujarat*			*Telangana*			*All*
	Sitamarhi	*Samastipur*	*Total*	*Sabarkantha*	*Dahod*	*Total*	*Medak*	*Vikarabad*	*Total*	
Self-employed (agriculture)	18.78	25.47	22.00	76.35	78.64	77.51	76.62	87.06	81.84	59.35
Self-employed (agriculture)	9.61	2.83	6.35	2.46	6.80	4.65	7.96	0.00	3.98	5.03
Regular wage earners	51.09	41.98	46.71	2.96	0.97	1.96	5.47	6.97	6.22	19.09
Casual labour (agriculture)	14.41	14.15	14.29	9.36	11.17	10.27	2.99	4.48	3.73	9.58
Casual labour (non-agriculture)	3.93	9.43	6.58	0.99	0.97	0.98	2.99	1.00	1.99	3.27
Government employment	0.44	0.00	0.23	0.00	0.00	0.00	0.00	0.00	0.00	0.08
Others	1.75	6.13	3.86	7.88	1.46	4.65	3.98	0.50	2.24	3.59
Total	100.00	100.00	100.00	100.00	100.00	100.00	100.00	100.00	100.00	100.00

Source: Own Primary Survey, 2018
Note: SE = Self-employed

in the Medak district of Telangana, agriculture is the major primary occupation. The principal crops produced were maize, paddy, and vegetables. In Lingampally village, the best-performing village in Vikarabad district of Telangana, villagers produced cotton, maize, paddy, millets, and vegetables as the main crops. The primary occupation of households in Allapur village, another best-performing village in Vikarabad, was producing cotton, maize, paddy, millets, and vegetables.

On the contrary, the primary occupation of inhabitants of Wadiyaram village, a worse-performing village in the same block, was livestock rearing. The primary occupation of the scheduled tribe (ST) community was piggery. Scheduled caste (SC) and other backward castes (OBC) households were primarily engaged in cattle rearing though all villages did not follow the same pattern. In the Neelapally village in Vikarabad, cotton, maize, paddy, millets, and vegetables were produced as the main crops.

The economic status of the households can be understood from per capita monthly expenditure. The average monthly per capita expenditure of survey households was Rs. 1439. The per capita expenditure was highest for the sample households from Bihar and lowest in Telangana (Figure 4.7). The per capita expenses of two Gujarat districts were on two ends. The per capita expenditure was much higher in the Sabarkantha district of Gujarat than in all other survey districts. On the contrary, the per capita household expenditure in the Dahod district of Gujarat was the lowest among the six districts under the survey.

Household Expenditure Pattern

The expenditure pattern of the households in all the three states was fascinating and provided a solid sense of expenditure priority at the family and community levels. The percentage of expenditure for various household requirements reveals that households in Telangana spent about 17% of total expenditure on food, which was

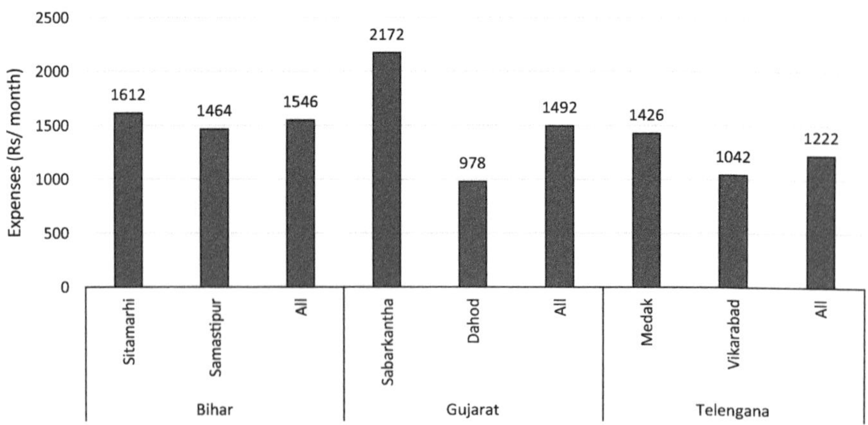

Figure 4.7 Per Capita Total Expenses of the Survey Households.

Source: Primary Survey

less in comparison to the spending of households of Bihar and Gujarat (Table 4.7). The highest spending on food was reported in Gujarat at 38%. Households in Sabarkantha spent 42% on food consumption, while households in Samastipur and Vikarabad spent 17% on food. It is observed that the expenditure on medicine was more or less the same across the states. But if we go deeper into districts, we find that the households in Vikarabad spent only 5% on medicine.

In comparison, households in Dahod spent around 17% of the expenditure on medicine or medical facilities. Households in Bihar spent the least on education at 8% of total expenditure, while households in two other states, Gujarat and Telangana, spent 18% and 16%, respectively, on education. The community's poor access to education facilities might be one of the reasons for the low expenditure on education in Bihar. Expenditure on food, medicine, and education accounted for about 70% of expenditure among surveyed households in Gujarat of their total expendable budget. In comparison, households of the other two states spent less than 45%.

Households in Bihar spent minimally on clothing and cosmetics at 6%, while households in Telangana spent around 24% on clothing and cosmetics. However, households in Bihar spent around half on durable goods like bicycles, motorcycles, television, mobile, etc. The expenditure on durable goods was the lowest in Gujarat. Construction of toilets, especially with own resources, may be compared with purchasing durable goods. The expenditure pattern implies that households in Bihar were more likely to spend on toilet construction. The state government's ban on alcohol consumption diverted money to toilet construction, as opined by male and female community members. On the other hand, households in Gujarat were less likely to spend on the toilet as they spent the most on essential food and education.

Dwelling Facility of the Households

The dwelling space of the household has an important bearing on the accessibility and availability of sanitation. Therefore, we attempted to understand the status of the households' dwellings. Space and ownership of the land play an important role in availing of any sanitation facility within the residential premise. About 97% of the total sample households owned a residential house. The residential house might be an ancestral property purchased or constructed by family members. Only 2% of the households lived in a rented house or with their relatives. Almost every household in the village had their own independent house (97.36%) rather than flat or other kinds of arrangement. Owned residences and independent houses make it easier to construct toilets if the households desire them.

The construction material of the house has implications on the general living standard of the households and, therefore, their propensity to use the toilet. The construction materials varied across states as well as districts. Materials like mud, grass, straw, leaves, reeds, bamboo, and cloth are considered *Katcha* or non-permanent structures. On the other hand, materials like burnt brick, stone, limestone, cement, reinforced brick concrete, reinforced cement concrete, etc. are considered

Table 4.7 Percentage Distribution of Expenditure by Items

Expenditure Items	*Bihar*			*Gujarat*			*Telangana*			*All*
	Sitamarhi	*Samastipur*	*Total*	*Sabarkantha*	*Dahod*	*Total*	*Medak*	*Vikarabad*	*Total*	
Food	28.00	17.67	22.31	42.03	24.34	37.81	20.43	17.80	16.51	32.75
Medicine	13.91	11.43	12.38	10.41	17.67	13.08	16.94	4.87	12.12	17.64
Education	8.33	7.38	7.64	21.34	16.73	18.07	30.66	9.17	16.21	16.44
Clothing and cosmetics	6.93	5.68	6.16	12.62	19.35	14.83	20.68	30.12	23.81	14.98
Durable goods	42.83	57.85	51.51	13.60	21.90	16.21	11.29	38.04	31.35	18.19
Total	100.00	100.00	100.00	100.00	100.00	100.00	100.00	100.00	100.00	100.00

Source: Own Primary Survey, 2018

Pucca or permanent construction. It is observed that a much higher proportion of households in Bihar had *Katcha* floor, wall, and roof as compared to other states (Table 4.8). The construction material of survey households in Telangana was better than that of other states.

Grass, straw, leaves, reeds, bamboo, etc. were generally used to construct the wall of the dwelling in Bihar, while in Telangana, cement, RBC, and RCC were used to construct the wall of the dwelling. The use of unburnt bricks was highest in Gujarat. About 45% of the households of Dahod used unburnt mud brick to construct the dwelling wall. About 72% of the households of Dahod had other types of kutcha roofs made up of unburnt mud brick and used asbestos for the roof of the dwelling. During the field visits in Dahod, it was observed that many households were engaged in manufacturing mud bricks in the brick factory in the locality. However, the disparity of construction materials across districts was stark within the state. About 61% of the households in Sabarkantha built the house's roof with cement, RBC, RCC, etc.

Access to Basic Services

We have enquired about access to essential services such as kitchen, drinking water, bathroom, and housing type. This information provided us with insights into the overall living standard of the households. Access to these services is supposed to have implications for access to toilets.

Kitchen Type

Many households did not have a separate kitchen (64%); they had to cook in commonplace or the passage. During the field visits, it was observed that few households were cooking in the bedroom because they did not have any other space for cooking. The majority of the households were using commonplace passages for bathing or cooking. Everyday use of the space for cooking, bathing, and cleaning is inconvenient and concerning due to the potential of spreading bacteria and germs through food to the human body. Within the three states, the percentage of households having no separate space for a kitchen was highest in Bihar at 85%. The intra-district divergence regarding access to the kitchen was very stark. Sabarkantha was the only district where more than 30% of households had a separate kitchen and tap water facility. In comparison, only 2% of households in Dahod had a separate kitchen with a tap.

The type of material used for the kitchen also reveals the standard of living of the households. About 50% of households in Gujarat had kitchens made of brick and mortar (permanent structure). The surveyed villages of Telangana and Bihar had permanent structures only in 30% and 7% of households, respectively. In Bihar, about 86% of households had mud structures for kitchens. Most households did not have a separate place to cook; instead, they used the commonplace for cooking in their mud thatched houses. The type of kitchen was observed to be best in Sabarkantha, where 70% of households had a permanent kitchen of brick and mortar.

Table 4.8 Percentage Distribution of Households by Construction Materials

Material Type	*Materials*	*Bihar*			*Gujarat*			*Telangana*			*All*		
		Floor	*Wall*	*Roof*	*Floor*	*Wall*	*Roof*	*Floor*	*Wall*	*Roof*	*Floor*	*Wall*	*Roof*
Katcha	Grass/straw/leaves/reeds/bamboo, etc.	0.68	48.75	59.09	4.65	1.22	2.69	1	0.75	5	2.08	17.81	23.3
	Mud/unburnt brick	86.39	21.54	5	28.36	31.05	6.85	20.15	29.85	5.75	46.17	27.32	5.84
	Other Katcha	0	0.23	0.46	0	4.89	37.41	0	0.25	1.25	0	1.76	12.81
Pucca	Tiles/slate		0.68	0		1.71	0.49		0.75	32.75		1.04	10.65
	Burnt brick/stone/limestone	3.85	15.19	2.27	11	40.34	9.78	48.01	3.48	25.25	20.37	19.65	12.09
	Iron/zinc/other metal sheet/asbestos sheet		1.36	5.91		0.24	4.65		0.25	1.75		0.64	4.16
	Cement/RBC/RCC	7.26	11.11	26.14	48.9	20.29	37.65	29.1	64.68	26.75	27.88	31.31	30.1
	Other Pucca	1.81	1.13	1.14	7.09	0.24	0.49	1.75	0	1.5	3.52	0.48	1.04
	Total	100	100	100	100	100	100	100	100	100	100	100	100

Source: Own Primary Survey, 2018

Households' Access to Water

The principal source of drinking water in all the three states differed and even varied among the districts of the same state. Overall, there were two significant sources of drinking water: tube well or borewell and piped water supply (Table 4.9). In Bihar, most households used tube wells or borewells. A quarter of the households used public standpoint in Samastipur while only 10% in Sitamarhi. In the Sabarkantha district of Gujarat, three-fourths of the households had access to piped water supply. But in the Dahod district, around half of the households used tube wells and around 40% used unprotected wells, which are potential causes of health hazards. In Telangana, most households used protected sources to access drinking water, which was true for about three-fourths of the households in Vikarabad. In Telangana, Mission Bhagiratha was launched to deliver a safe and sustainable piped water supply to every household. However, in Medak, 65% of households were found collecting water from nearby water stations.

Households used bottled water to access safe water in Sabarkantha and Samastipur. Arsenic and fluoride contamination was one of the significant concerns in the Samastipur district. Moreover, there was the problem of water availability throughout the year. Households purchased bottles containing 20 litres of water for Rs. 20. Households in Bihar could not afford bottled water for drinking and other household chores even when they were aware of the high level of arsenic and fluoride in water. The people of Dahod lived a difficult life due to a lack of water availability and accessibility. But still, bottled water purchase was low due to the inability to pay.

Recent government initiatives made safe water available to the doorsteps of people. Implementing Mission Bhagiratha by the Telangana state government helped the community with the timely availability of water in their dwelling in Telangana villages. However, we observed that the households of Medak were highly dependent on bottled water as the principal source of drinking instead of piped water. There were two main reasons: one, poor connectivity and availability of water under Mission Bhagiratha in the villages of Medak; and two, water stations installed near Panchayat by the Safe Water Network were far away from many households. The Safe Water Network operates through small water enterprises (SWEs) to ensure the delivery of safe and reliable drinking water. *iJal* Safe Water Stations were constructed as a water purifier machine in the village with 24×7 water availability. *iJal* Safe Water Stations were locally owned and operated as small water enterprises (SWEs). Villagers were trained to use the water vending machine by swapping debit cards provided by the organisation. Due to water availability through *iJal* Safe Water Stations, bottled water was cheaper in Telangana than in Bihar. A 20-litre bottle used to cost Rs. 5 in Medak while it was Rs. 20 in Samastipur. Overall, Mission Bhagiratha provided better access to water supply in Telangana than the other two states.

Water sources for exclusive household use were available for 65% of the households. The same was as high as 96% in Telangana, primarily due to Mission Bhagiratha. It includes bottled water and water from the water station. On the other

Table 4.9 Percentage Distribution of Households by Principal Source of Drinking Water Supply

	Bihar			*Gujarat*			*Telangana*			*All*
Source	*Sitamarhi*	*Samastipur*	*Total*	*Sabarkantha*	*Dahod*	*Total*	*Medak*	*Vikarabad*	*Total*	
Bottled water/ water station	0.0	4.2	2.0	9.4	1.5	5.4	65.2	0.5	32.8	13.0
Piped water into dwelling	1.7	7.1	4.3	76.4	1.9	38.9	27.9	74.1	51.0	30.6
Piped water to yard/plot	0.4	0.5	0.5	1.0	0.0	0.5	0.5	1.0	0.7	0.6
Public tap/stand pipe	9.6	24.1	16.6	0.5	0.0	0.2	1.0	3.5	2.2	6.6
Tube well/ borehole	88.2	61.8	75.5	3.9	47.6	25.9	5.0	20.9	12.9	39.2
Well protected	0.0	0.0	0.0	0.5	10.7	5.6	0.0	0.0	0.0	1.8
Well unprotected	0.0	0.0	0.0	0.0	38.3	19.3	0.0	0.0	0.0	6.3
Others (tank/ pond/stream/ river)	0.0	2.4	1.1	8.4	0.0	4.2	0.5	0.0	0.2	1.8
Total	100	100	100	100	100	100	100	100	100	100
Availability of water sufficient throughout the year (%)	86.46	74.06	80.50	89.16	98.54	93.89	96.52	92.04	94.28	89.30

Source: Own Primary Survey, 2018

hand, access to exclusive household use was deficient in Dahod (Table 4.10). Only 2% of the households in Dahod had drinking water facilities within their dwelling. Moreover, 44% of the households had to carry water from 200 meters, and 46% had to carry water from more than 200 meters.

Bathing Space

It is essential to understand the overall picture of accessibility and availability of proper bathing space to understand the sanitation facility at the grassroots. About half of the rural households surveyed did not have any bathrooms. Most took baths in the open or a shared space within the house, near a tube well, in the backyard, or in the passage or corridor of the house. Around 80% of Bihar households had no bathrooms (Table 4.11). On the other hand, households accessing a bathroom detached from their dwellings were highest in Telangana at 73%, about 92% of the households in the Medak district had detached bathrooms, and only 4% of households in the district had attached bathrooms in the dwellings. The intra-district variation was also wide. While only 4% of households in Medak district did not have a bathroom, the same was at 45% in Vikarabad. However, in Gujarat, the situation was different. Sabarkantha and Dahod districts had about 66% and 17% of households with attached bathrooms, respectively. In Sabarkantha and Dahod, 19% and 70% of the households had no bathrooms, respectively. When households had access to the bathroom, attached or detached, around 85% were for the exclusive use of the household. It also signifies the importance of bathrooms for exclusive use. However, aberration is observed in Gujarat, where around only 30% of households had access to a bathroom in their building. The same type of common access was available for 44% of households in Dahod. When households use the shared bathroom, they may also be able to use the shared toilet.

Gender and Water

It is also essential to understand the gender role in fetching the water for drinking and other domestic chores at the household level. Women are primarily responsible for reproductive and household chores. Fetching water for drinking and other household activities is an essential task that the household members, especially women, must perform. A distant water source may have implications on women's workload. Women were primarily responsible for fetching drinking water if the sources were outside their premises. Among households whose sources of drinking water supply were outside the premises, in around 70% households women above 18 years were fetching water (Table 4.12). The same holds for more than 90% of households in Gujarat and 80% of households in Bihar. The most concerning fact was that 36% of females aged less than 18 years used to fetch water from outside premises in the Sabarkantha district of Gujarat. Whereas, in Telangana, a substantial percentage of male members fetched drinking water. The same was highest in the Medak district, where in 63% of households, males above 18 years used to

Table 4.10 Percentage Distribution of Households by Type of Access and Distance of Primary Source of Drinking Water

		Bihar			*Gujarat*			*Telangana*			*All*
		Sitamarhi	*Samastipur*	*Total*	*Sabarkantha*	*Dahod*	*Total*	*Medak*	*Vikarabad*	*Total*	
Type of access	Household's exclusive use	66.81	65.69	65.08	64.53	3.4	33.74	96.52	95.02	95.77	64.7
	Common use of households in the building	3.06	2.45	2.72	29.06	58.25	43.77	3.48	4.98	4.23	16.61
	Neighbour/ community/ public	29.25	30.39	29.25	2.46	21.36	11.98	0	0	0	14.22
	Others	0.87	1.47	2.94	3.94	16.99	10.51	0	0	0	4.47
	Total	100	100	100	100	100	100	100	100	100	100
Distance	Within dwelling	60.26	56.13	58.28	64.04	2.43	33.01	25.87	50.25	38.06	43.53
	Outside dwelling but within the premises	12.66	13.21	12.93	30.54	7.28	18.83	16.42	28.36	22.39	17.89
	Outside premises: less than 0.2 km	26.64	26.89	26.76	5.42	44.17	24.94	27.86	16.42	22.14	24.68
	Outside premises: more than 0.2 km	0.44	3.77	2.04	0	46.12	23.23	29.86	4.98	17.41	13.91
	Total	100	100	100	100	100	100	100	100	100	100

Source: Own Primary Survey, 2018

Table 4.11 Percentage Distribution of Households by Bathroom Availability and Type of Access

Access to Bathroom		*Bihar*			*Gujarat*			*Telangana*			*All*
		Sitamarhi	*Samastipur*	*Total*	*Sabarkantha*	*Dahod*	*Total*	*Medak*	*Vikarabad*	*Total*	
Availability of bathroom	Attached	20.09	20.75	20.41	66.01	17.48	41.56	3.98	0.5	2.24	21.49
	Detached	0.87	1.89	1.36	15.27	13.11	14.18	92.04	54.23	73.13	28.59
	No bathroom	79.04	77.36	78.23	18.72	69.42	44.25	3.98	45.27	24.63	49.92
	Total	100	100	100	100	100	100	100	100	100	100
Type of access	Exclusive use of household	97.96	88.24	93.00	72.73	55.56	67.98	90.82	98.20	93.49	84.25
	Common use of households in the building	2.04	9.80	6.00	26.06	44.44	31.14	7.65	0.90	5.21	14.65
	Public/ community use/others	0.00	1.96	1.00	1.21	0.00	0.88	1.53	0.90	1.30	1.10
	Total	100	100	100	100	100	100	100	100	100	100

Source: Own Primary Survey, 2018

Table 4.12 Percentage Distribution of Households by Members/Non-Members Responsible to Fetch Drinking Water

Responsibility	*Bihar*			*Gujarat*			*Telangana*			*All*
	Sitamarhi	*Samastipur*	*Total*	*Sabarkantha*	*Dahod*	*Total*	*Medak*	*Vikarabad*	*Total*	
Male of age below 18 years	6.12	3.74	4.88	0.00	0.00	0.00	2.13	0.64	1.45	1.98
Male of age 18 years and above	6.12	15.89	11.22	0.00	0.00	0.00	62.77	19.75	43.19	22.66
Female of age below 18 years	1.02	0.00	0.49	36.36	4.04	5.74	2.13	0.64	1.45	2.37
Female of age 18 years and above	85.71	76.64	80.98	63.64	95.45	93.78	20.21	78.34	46.67	68.91
Non-member/hired labour	1.02	3.74	2.44	0.00	0.51	0.48	12.77	0.64	7.25	4.08
Total	100	100	100	100	100	100	100	100	100	100

Source: Own Primary Survey, 2018

fetch water from outside. About 3% of households in the same district had non-members or hired labour fetching water.

Water for Household Chores

Water sources for household chores also had implications for women's workload. It had implications for access to water for the toilet as well. Sources within households may not increase the workload of women. If sources are outside the dwelling, either woman must fetch water or take the work to a distant water source. Non-availability of water can also create stress and may have negative implications for toilet use. The uses of water also varied. A substantial proportion of households' piped water supply was used for household cleaning (Table 4.13). However, this was held for districts of Telangana and only the Sabarkantha district of Gujarat. Households in Bihar depended on public tap to a large extent. Most of the households in Bihar and a substantial proportion of households in Dahod depended on tube wells for household cleaning. Furthermore, around 40% of households in Dahod used wells for household cleaning activities.

Water availability throughout the year for household cleaning and other household chores was insufficient for 9% of households (Table 4.13). The same problem was observed in Bihar, where 15% of households in Sitamarhi and around a quarter of the households in Samastipur had the same problem with water availability. Arsenic and fluoride contamination was the cause of distress in Bihar. Although almost all the households reported sufficient water availability in the Dahod district, the field visits provided the impression that there was an irregularity in water availability at household and community levels. Children in the community also shared the burden of fetching water from various sources such as a pond, tube well, etc. This lack of water availability would negatively affect toilet use in these districts.

Access to Toilet and Type of Toilet

Across states, about 53% of households had access to the toilets for exclusive use, while 34% had no access to the toilet. Access to the toilet was best in Telangana (76%), followed by Gujarat (65%) and Bihar (59%). There was considerable variation among the states and districts regarding the type of toilet used. While access to the toilet for exclusive use was highest in Telangana, followed by Bihar, access to the standard toilet was better in Gujarat than in other states. Among all other districts, Medak of Telangana was the only district which showed that more than 90% of HHs had access to the toilet exclusively used. Following Medak, in the Sitamarhi district of Bihar, 72% of households had a toilet for exclusive use. Districts with low coverage of toilets were the Vikarabad district of Telangana, Dahod district of Gujarat, and Samastipur district of Bihar (Table 4.14).

Among various toilets, 60% were toilets with a septic tank, and only 12% were pit toilets (Table 4.15). The states show a wide variation in pit toilets vis-à-vis the septic tank toilets. Both the districts of Telangana registered the highest number of septic tank toilets (90%), compared to Bihar (58%) and Gujarat (22%). Pit toilet

Table 4.13 Percentage Distribution of Households Source of Water Supply for Household Chores and Availability of Water

		Bihar			*Gujarat*			*Telangana*			*All*
		Sitamarhi	*Samastipur*	*Total*	*Sabarkantha*	*Dahod*	*Total*	*Medak*	*Vikarabad*	*Total*	
Sources	Piped water into dwelling	1.75	4.25	2.95	78.82	3.88	41.08	96.02	95.02	95.52	45.13
	Piped water to yard/plot	0.44	0.94	0.68	0.99	0.49	0.73	0	1	0.5	0.64
	Public tap/ standpipe	34.93	38.68	36.73	0.99	7.77	4.4	1	0.5	0.75	14.62
	Tube well/ borehole	62.45	53.77	58.28	4.93	41.75	23.47	1	2.99	1.99	28.83
	Well	0.44	0	0.23	0	39.32	19.8	0	0	0	6.55
	Surface water: tank/ponds	0	0	0	9.85	0	4.89	0	0	0	1.6
	Other sources	0	2.36	1.13	4.42	6.79	5.63	1.98	0.49	1.24	2.63
	Total	100	100	100	100	100	100	100	100	100	100
Water sufficiently available throughout the year (%)		84.72	76.42	80.73	89.16	99.03	94.13	99	98.51	98.76	90.89

Source: Own Primary Survey, 2018

Table 4.14 Percentage Distribution of Households by Access to Toilet and Type of Toilet Used

		Bihar			*Gujarat*			*Telangana*			*All*
		Sitamarhi	*Samastipur*	*Total*	*Sabarkantha*	*Dahod*	*Total*	*Medak*	*Vikarabad*	*Total*	
Access to toilet	Exclusive use of household	72.49	38.86	56.36	54.95	7.80	31.20	90.95	54.50	72.68	53.37
	Common use of households in the building	1.75	2.84	2.27	28.22	38.54	33.42	5.03	0.50	2.76	12.60
	Public/ community toilet	0.00	0.47	0.23	0.50	0.98	0.74	0.50	0.00	0.25	0.40
	No toilet	25.76	57.82	41.14	16.34	52.68	34.64	3.52	45.00	24.31	33.63
	Total	100	100	100	100	100	100	100	100	100	100
Type of toilet used	Flush/pour-flush to: piped sewer system	0.00	3.41	1.17	30.57	1.03	19.29	1.01	0.00	0.64	6.57
	Toilet with septic tank	63.10	47.73	57.81	29.30	9.28	21.65	92.96	95.58	93.91	60.34
	Pit toilet	0.60	9.09	3.52	29.94	43.30	35.04	0.50	0.00	0.32	12.04
	Ring type	18.45	22.73	19.92	0.00	0.00	0.00	0.00	0.00	0.00	6.20
	Others	17.86	14.77	16.80	0.64	3.09	1.57	4.52	4.42	4.49	7.42
	Not used (all members)	0.00	2.27	0.78	9.55	43.30	22.44	1.01	0.00	0.64	7.42
	Total	100.00	100.00	100.00	100.00	100.00	100.00	100.00	100.00	100.00	100.00

Source: Own Primary Survey, 2018

Table 4.15 Percentage of Households Where All Members Use Toilet If Having Access

Member Type	*Bihar*			*Gujarat*			*Telangana*			*All*
	Sitamarhi	*Samastipur*	*Total*	*Sabarkantha*	*Dahod*	*Total*	*Medak*	*Vikarabad*	*Total*	
Male below 15 years	91.77	95.89	93.07	96.49	90.57	94.61	92.39	91.94	92.21	93.30
Male above 15 years	93.41	96.67	94.55	97.95	96.36	97.51	93.75	100.00	96.00	95.91
Female below 15 years	90.63	88.73	90.04	97.09	90.38	94.84	91.58	92.42	91.93	91.96
Female above 15 years	96.43	96.70	96.53	94.70	92.73	94.17	96.39	100.00	97.68	96.35
Old aged (above 60 years)	38.14	70.54	55.50	32.04	9.09	26.47	80.00	5.88	22.73	42.78
All members	56.74	68.94	61.94	50.96	45.61	49.53	89.85	80.00	86.22	67.82

Source: Own Primary Survey, 2018

was more prevalent in Gujarat than the septic tank toilet. Flush or pour-flush toilet with piped sewer system was also maximum in Gujarat at 19%, particularly in the Sabarkantha district.

During the focus group discussions in Bihar and Telangana, it came to the surface that people believed that small soak pits might pollute and contaminate the groundwater; therefore, there was a lesser number of pit toilets in these two states. They believed that the soak pits were more hazardous than the open defecation. Because of the notions of purity and pollution, people did not like the idea of emptying the pit by themselves. Households prefer a septic tank because of its low-cost maintenance and no need to empty it in the future. Gujarat had the highest percentage of pit toilets compared to the other two states. Dahod had the maximum number of twin pit toilets among the other districts. During the field visits, we observed that the quality of the pit dug was very poor; it did not match the details mentioned in the SBM guidelines. In the Dahod district of Gujarat, 44% of the households were not using toilets despite having access. The quality of the pit could be one of the reasons for the low usage of toilets.

The government, NGOs, and many international organisations were promoting twin pit toilets, especially in rural areas. Field visits in the villages provided the information that organisations like JEEViKA, Aga Khan Foundation, UNICEF, Anarde Foundation, etc. had promoted the twin pit toilet at the grassroots. The main reason for promoting such a toilet was that the content of human excreta could be easily converted into manure with the help of a Y-section design. Table 4.15 reflects that only 12% of the households had constructed the pit toilet, while 60% had constructed the septic tank toilet. Toilet with the septic tank was most prevalent in Telangana. The main reason for constructing a septic tank in the villages was that the households were wary about pollution and purity. They believed that the smaller soak pits might pollute the groundwater and further decrease the quality of drinking water in the locality. They also felt that soak pits were more hazardous than open defecation. Another concern of the households was with emptying the septic tank. Most households prefer septic tanks as they needn't worry about filling the pit in their lifetime. Dahod had a maximum number of twin pit toilets among the other districts. At the same time, it was also observed during the field visits that the quality of pit dug was very poor and was not aligned with the details mentioned in the guideline. Poor infrastructure was the prime reason that 44% of households did not use toilets in the district.

Toilet Use

A toilet in residence is meant to be used for the purpose for which it is constructed. But, many households have constructed toilets that they may not use. Suppose a household has built a toilet under public sanitation programme where they made a minimal contribution. In that case, there is a higher probability that they may not use it as it lacks an individual household-level stake in the asset created. They may not be able to realise the benefits of using the toilet. If the social infrastructure such as easy access to water supply and household infrastructure such as the exclusive bathroom are not available, then the household may not use the toilet even if it is constructed and they have already contributed to it. The household may treat it as a sunk cost and would like to find an alternative use for the toilet, like storing fodder for their animals.

Our analysis of toilet use by different members of households demonstrates that in more than 90% of households, all members below 60 years of age used the toilet if they had access to it (Table 4.15). However, in only around 43% of households, all the older members above 60 years of age used the toilet. Interestingly, in Vikarabad, all males and females aged more than 15 years used toilets, but in only 6% of households, all old members used toilets. This type of disparity implies that the practice of open defecation was difficult to reverse for the old aged. Social norms may have played a spoilsport in ushering a behavioural change. The disparity of toilet use among members of different age groups defeats the idea of total sanitation. Only in 68% of households do all members use the toilet. All household members should use the toilet if they have to get the full health benefits of improved sanitation practices. Privacy and convenience might have influenced the adoption of improved sanitation behaviour. All male and female members above 15 years of age in most households used the toilet if they had access. However, what is concerning was that all female members aged less than 15 years in 8% of households did not use the toilet, which may have a negative impact on future adoption of improved sanitation behaviour.

Sanitation Facility Outside Dwelling

Workplaces, schools, and other commonplaces also need proper sanitation facilities for improved sanitation behaviour. At the same time, around 70% of the households revealed that they did not have at least one member of households having any sanitation facility in their workplace, and 7% of households reported that at least one member had a toilet at the workplace. Still, they did not have access to it (Table 4.16). Access to the toilet at the workplace was highest in Bihar and nil in Telangana, as access to a toilet at the household level was worst in Bihar and best in Telangana. The inter-district variation is also very high. While 92% of households in Dahod did not have at least one toilet at the workplace, 40% of households in Sabarkantha had at least one member having access to the toilet.

Access to the toilet at the school for children was very high, which would have a positive impact in the long run in terms of both sanitation behaviour and health outcomes. School toilet access was worse in Gujarat, especially in the Dahod district. Bihar, which was lagging in toilet access and other indicators of access to services, became one of the forerunners in children's toilet access at school.

Household-Level Health and Hygiene

The basic health and hygiene of the households may have implications for sanitation behaviour. Households with better health and hygiene conditions are more likely to practice improved sanitation. The survey results reveal that a substantial proportion of households was affected; at least one of the household members

Table 4.16 Distribution of Households by Access to Toilet at Workplace and School (in %)

		Bihar			*Gujarat*			*Telangana*			*All*
		Sitamarhi	*Samastipur*	*Total*	*Sabarkantha*	*Dahod*	*Total*	*Medak*	*Vikarabad*	*Total*	
Access at workplace	Yes, accessible	54	46	50	40	3	20	1	0	0	25
	No, have toilet but not accessible	4	10	7	19	5	12	5	1	3	7
	Do not have toilet at all	42	43	42	41	92	68	94	99	97	68
	Total	100	100	100	100	100	100	100	100	100	100
Access by children at school (%)		98	99	99	84	79	81	99	100	100	93

Source: Own Primary Survey, 2018

was affected by fever and stomach problems during the previous 30 days of the survey. The stomach problem was predominant in Bihar. The bad quality of water may be responsible for such degraded health conditions. Fever (other than malaria) was more prevalent in Telangana than in the other two states. The hygiene condition of the survey villages also captured the household's perception regarding the problem of mosquitoes and flies. The problem of mosquitoes and flies was primarily observed in Bihar. Households of Sitamarhi district reported the severeness of mosquito and fly menace. As discussed earlier, it may have caused other health-related problems in the state. Medak district of Telangana had the least problem with mosquitoes and flies. Although more than 50% of the sample households were suffering from severe issues of mosquitoes and flies in all the three states, 64% of the total survey households reported that there was no preventive and curative action by the local governments such as PRIs or state governments during the last one year to the survey. On the other hand, 56% of the total survey households reported that though the local bodies did not take action, the households tried to resolve the issues of mosquitoes and flies at their level. Measures like spray, coil, mosquito-killing mat, burning of the bush, and using kerosene oil and mosquito net were the few actions the community or households took.

Summary and Conclusion

We have conducted an in-depth survey in three states of India: Bihar, Gujarat, and Telangana. These three states belong to three different cultural zones defined by the Government of India. Moreover, the coverage of toilets in the three states is varied. The best- and worst-performing districts and blocks were selected from these three states to make the sample representative. In total, 1252 sample households were surveyed with the help of a pre-designed questionnaire. A qualitative study was conducted through in-depth structured and unstructured interviews. Participatory Rural Appraisal (PRA was conducted to understand the households' perception of their social environment and availability of social infrastructure and resources. Zaltman Metaphor Elicitation Technique (Z-MET) was used to understand the user's perspective of sanitation.

The respondents of the survey were primarily heads of households. On average, there were six members per household. In 21% of households, all male members and in 35% of households, all female members were illiterate. More than 90% of households were Hindu, and only 7% were upper (general) castes. Around 60% of households were self-employed in agriculture, while around 20% were regular wage or salaried persons. The per capita average monthly expenditure, an indicator of the economic well-being of households, was Rs. 1439. The economic condition of households appears to be best in Gujarat and worst in Bihar. However, there was wide variation across districts within a state. While the economic condition of survey households in Sabarkantha district appeared to be the best, the same for households in the Dahod district of Gujarat was the worst among all the study districts. The expenditure paper of households, which depicts their economic condition and priority, varied across states. The households mainly spent on necessities like food, medicine, and education.

The basic living condition of the households depicts their economic condition and standard of living. Almost all the households used to reside in their owned dwellings. Almost half of the dwellings had their floor and wall made of *Katcha* materials, while most had roofs made of *Pucca*. Around 65% of households within the dwelling did not have a separate kitchen. Primary water sources for drinking and other household chores were tube wells or borewells followed by household piped water. The access to the sources was exclusive for the household in 65% of the cases. More than 60% of the sources were within the premises. Adult women were primarily responsible for fetching water. Half of the households did not have access to the bathroom.

A substantial percentage of households did not have access to a toilet at the time of the survey. While 34% of the respondents had no toilet access, it was highest in Samastipur (58%). Overall, the coverage was best in Telangana and worst in Bihar. Interestingly, despite the government sanitation programme advocating for pit toilets, only 12% of households had the same. Moreover, the Dahod district, where the prevalence of pit toilets was the highest, also had the highest percentage of households not using the toilet. Around 68% of households did not have any household member who had a toilet at their workplace. However, children generally had access to a toilet at school.

The lack of availability of toilets affected the health of the households as a substantial proportion of them suffered stomach problems, fever, and malaria in recent times. The nuisance of mosquitoes and flies affected almost 90% of the survey households. Overall, this chapter illustrates fundamental infrastructure problems at the household level. The economic condition of the households was also constrained. Under these circumstances, a large proportion of households was yet to get access to a toilet. The government sanitation programme advocated pit toilets, but the basic design and construction material discouraged people from using them.

Notes

1 https://www.indiaculture.nic.in/about-us/autonomus-bodies/zonal-cultural-centers.
2 The survey was conducted in June–September of 2018.

5 Toilet Construction and Behavioural Change

The decision of individuals regarding the use of toilets is crucially dependent on their attitude towards sanitation and practices in society. On the one hand, human behaviour can be influenced by personal normative beliefs, which are personal beliefs about what should one do (Bicchieri, 2016). On the other hand, people's behaviour may be influenced by their environment. People may follow what others do, irrespective of what others want them to do. This kind of collective behaviour is a descriptive norm. People may follow others not only as others practice some behaviour but also as others expect them to follow what they do. The latter type of collective behaviour is social norms. These different types of collective behaviours form the environment under which a person decides their sanitation behaviour. Hence, it is crucial to understand individual attitudes and the environment, which may influence a person's sanitation behaviour.

To understand the importance given by households for toilet use, we have investigated the personal priority and timing of toilet construction. If the construction has taken place during the construction of the house, then the household has given more priority to toilet construction. We have also investigated the direct reasons for toilet construction and not constructing and using toilets to understand factors that form people's attitudes towards sanitation. We have also examined the sanitation environment by examining their awareness regarding sanitation, public health campaigns, public initiatives to make them aware and encourage toilet construction, and other sources from which they might have been influenced to construct a toilet.

Toilet Construction: Priority and Timing

One of the least investigated aspects of sanitation behaviour is the timing of construction. When constructing the house, whether the owner or the head of the household had contemplated the necessity of having a toilet or not would reveal the household's priority for having a toilet. Thus, it is essential to analyse the timing of the construction of the toilet. Generally, the households that plan to construct the house have a blueprint in mind to accommodate various priorities given the constraints of space and money. When sanitation is one of the priorities of the household, then the household would plan and construct at the time of construction of the house itself. The household will construct it later if it is not one of the top

DOI: 10.4324/9781032726267-5

priorities during construction. Our survey reveals that in the case of most households, the toilet was not one of the household's priorities at the time of construction of the house. Only 14% of households had constructed a toilet during the time of house construction, while 53% of the households had constructed it later. Toilet constructed at the time of the house was the highest in Gujarat but with very high variation amongst districts. Sabarkantha villages had about 50% of the households that constructed toilets during the house construction, but in Dahod, only 3% had contemplated having a toilet. Among the districts, 85% of household toilets in Medak and around 70% of household toilets in Sitamarhi were constructed later.

Government sanitation campaigns might have encouraged households to construct toilets later over the years. Overall, about 46% of the households had constructed their toilet within ten years of the construction of the house (Table 5.1). Among the districts, households in Dahod appear to be the fastest to construct toilets after the construction of the house. Half of the households in Dahod constructed toilets within five years of construction, and 95% constructed toilets within ten years of house construction. In contrast, only 17% of households constructed toilets within ten years of house construction in the Medak district. Launching a government sanitation programme around house construction may have played a significant role in such a pattern.

Our analysis reveals that most toilets were constructed much after the house construction during the Swachh Bharat Mission (SBM), i.e., after 2015. Bihar has been very slow in picking up sanitation and showed impressive toilet construction. In our sample households from Bihar, Gujarat, and Telangana, about 89%, 80%, and 59% of the households had their toilets constructed after 2015, respectively, which was long after the construction of their residences, which implies that SBM significantly impacts toilet construction in all three states, especially Bihar and Gujarat. Toilet construction picked up between 2010 and 2015 in the Medak district of Telangana and the Sabarkantha district in Gujarat (Figure 5.1). These districts were the early adopters of improved sanitation behaviour when TSC, followed by NBA, was in operation.

Although a more significant number of toilets were constructed recently, many were not constructed under SBM. This indicated that SBM might have an indirect impact on toilet construction. Toilets were constructed with their resources or supported by sources other than SBM. For example, in Neelapalle village in Vikarabad district of Telangana 25 toilets were constructed, out of which 7 were constructed under the Mahatma Gandhi National Rural Employment Guarantee Act 2005 (MGNREGA), and 18 toilets were constructed under SBM.

Our survey revealed that among those who do not have a toilet in all three states, more than 95% of households were willing to construct a toilet in the future. However, the willingness was lesser at 86% in Sabarkantha and Medak districts. While enquiring about when households would construct a toilet in the future, 74% did not have any definite plan. The same was very high in Telangana, followed by Bihar (Figure 5.2). In Gujarat, 25% of households decided to construct toilets within the next six months. Overall, 20% of households decided to construct toilets within a year. The analysis implies that households may not have long-term

Table 5.1 Percentage of Households by Reasons for Toilet Construction

Reasons for Constructing Toilets	*Bihar*			*Gujarat*			*Telangana*			*All*
	Sitamarhi	*Samastipur*	*Total*	*Sabarkantha*	*Dahod*	*Total*	*Medak*	*Vikarabad*	*Total*	
Privacy	70.31	34.43	53.06	28.57	37.38	33.01	31.84	30.35	31.09	39.46
Convenience	52.40	29.25	41.27	79.80	38.35	58.92	36.82	20.40	28.61	42.97
Potential health benefits	50.66	27.83	39.68	10.84	33.50	22.25	34.33	3.48	18.91	27.32
Other important reason	13.97	6.13	10.20	5.42	4.85	5.13	2.49	0.00	1.24	5.67
Benefits from govt. subsidy	2.18	0.94	1.59	0.99	1.46	1.22	2.49	0.50	1.49	1.44
Forced/coercion by officials/ leaders	0.44	2.36	1.36	0.99	0.00	0.49	6.97	3.98	5.47	2.40
Peer pressure and prestige in the society	0.44	1.89	1.13	3.45	0.00	1.71	9.45	7.46	8.46	3.67
Not applicable	25.76	57.55	41.04	16.75	52.43	34.72	3.98	45.27	24.63	33.71
Total	100.00	100.00	100.00	100.00	100.00	100.00	100.00	100.00	100.00	100.00

Source: Own Primary Survey, 2018

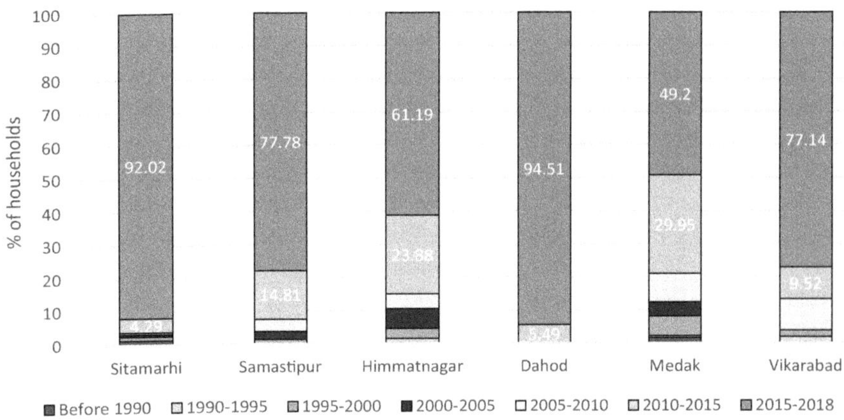

Figure 5.1 Construction of Toilet after House Construction.

Source: Own Primary Survey, 2018

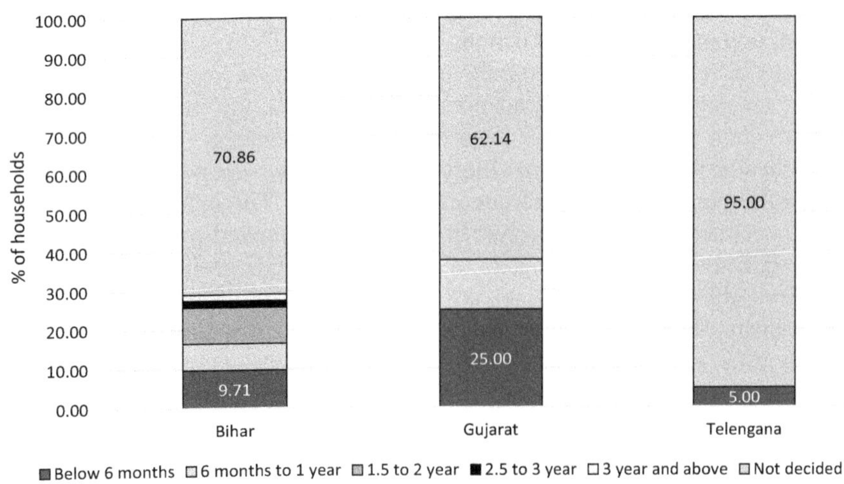

Figure 5.2 Plan for Toilet Construction Within Specific Time.

Source: Primary Data (Authors)

planning for toilet construction. If they decided to construct within a time frame, then it would be within the next year.

Reasons for Construction of Toilet

During the survey, we asked the households explicitly the major reasons for toilet construction. Households have given multiple reasons for toilet construction, which provides insights into significant drivers of behaviour change in sanitation. Convenience and privacy were the most common reasons for constructing the toilets in the households. Potential health benefits due to toilet construction emerged as the third important reason. In Bihar, privacy was the most critical reason to construct a toilet, while in Gujarat, the convenience of using a toilet was more important. Households in Telangana gave almost equal importance to privacy and convenience (Table 5.1).

The potential health benefits were an essential driver of toilet construction in Bihar, where 40% of households constructed toilets due to potential health benefits. The households giving importance to potential health benefits were highest in the Sitamarhi district. It may be due to problems regarding health and hygiene in the district. Malaria affected 20% of households; the severe problem of mosquitoes and flies was reported by 98% of households, and 56% of households suffered from stomach problems in Sitamarhi. Moreover, malaria and other types of fever severely affected households in Medak and Dahod districts. About 42% of households in Medak and 34% in Dahod were affected by fever during the last month of the survey.

On top of that, 18% of households in Dahod were affected by malaria. These health issues may have driven households in Medak and Dahod to construct toilets contemplating its potential health benefits. Hence, health and hygiene concerns are significant drivers of toilet construction.

We have directly enquired about the influences that have resulted in toilet construction. Overall, 44% of respondents reported that no one influenced them in the construction of the toilet, not even other family members (Table 5.2). They have decided on toilet construction. More than half of the respondents in Bihar and 45% in Telangana opined that no one influenced them. The influence of spouses in toilet construction is most decisive in Telangana, followed by Bihar. Children were the critical information carriers to their respective households. Children in Bihar were very aware of sanitation and cleanliness drives such as hand washing and Swacchata Abhiyan (clean campaign). The influence of school-going children, especially girls, and the influence of children above school-going age had a substantial impact on toilet construction in Gujarat. Furthermore, the influence of other household members was also highest in Gujarat.

The influence of local political leaders was observed to be highest in the Dahod district, and the influence of health and the social worker was the most in Medak. Peer pressure from neighbours or friends has played a very prominent role in Vikarabad. Hence, although self-motivation was the primary driver for toilet construction, the influence of other household members, especially children, neighbours, local political leaders, and health or social workers, also played a significant role. However, the primary sources of influence are different in different districts.

Government programmes may have benefitted the households by instigating a behaviour change, but there were concerns about applying force and coercion for toilet construction. It was mainly reported in Telangana, especially in Medak. Local political leaders threatened community members that if they did not construct toilets, they would be barred from availing the benefits of other government schemes such as public distribution system, pension, electricity, etc. Peer pressure is one of the critical driving forces for sanitation behaviour change worldwide,

Table 5.2 Percentage Distribution of Respondents by Sources of Influence for Toilet Construction

	Bihar			*Gujarat*			*Telangana*			*All*
	Sitamarhi	*Samastipur*	*Total*	*Sabarkantha*	*Dahod*	*Total*	*Medak*	*Vikarabad*	*Total*	
Self	63.75	37.58	53.09	40.80	27.80	35.78	51.56	35.25	45.33	43.85
Spouse	12.08	24.85	17.28	11.66	6.34	9.60	21.33	38.85	28.02	17.15
School-going male children	0.83	2.42	1.48	4.91	5.37	5.08	0.00	0.00	0.00	2.54
School-going female children	1.25	4.24	2.47	8.59	7.80	8.29	0.89	0.72	0.82	4.38
Children above school-going age	1.25	4.24	2.47	8.59	7.80	8.29	0.89	0.72	0.82	4.38
Elders	0.00	2.42	0.99	1.23	0.98	1.13	0.44	0.00	0.27	0.85
Other household members	5.42	12.12	8.15	13.50	24.88	17.89	2.67	5.04	3.57	10.85
Neighbours or Friends	3.75	1.21	2.72	1.84	2.44	2.07	2.22	10.79	5.49	3.23
Political or Panchayat leaders	4.17	4.24	4.20	6.13	14.15	9.23	1.33	1.44	1.37	5.46
Health or social worker	7.50	6.67	7.16	2.76	2.44	2.64	18.67	7.19	14.29	7.31
Total	100	100	100	100	100	100	100	100	100	100

Source: Own Primary Survey, 2018

but pressure by official or political leaders defeats the purpose of demand-driven behaviour change. The implementation of government programmes should consider that pressure from influential individuals should be avoided, although peer pressure is welcome.

Reasons for Not Constructing and Using Toilet

The primary reason for not constructing toilets was a lack of financial ability (Table 5.3). The same was why not constructing toilets in almost all Gujarat households. Not owning a house was one of the primary reasons for not constructing the toilet in Bihar. Lack of space in the dwelling was cited as one of the prominent reasons for not constructing a toilet in the Vikarabad district. It is important to note that the reason for not constructing toilets for 10% of Telangana households was that they could not perceive any benefit of toilet use. About 40% of Medak households did not have a particular reason for not constructing toilets. Households that do not find any motivation to construct toilets or do not have any significant reason for not constructing toilets should be motivated through government IEC programmes. Households that cannot construct toilets due to lack of availability of their land should be given access to community toilets. Households that could not construct toilets due to financial constraints should be better targeted under the public sanitation programme.

The economic constraint was a significant challenge for toilet construction, even under a public sanitation programme like SBM. It is because the government's incentive of Rs. 12000 for toilet construction is received by beneficiaries only after toilet construction. The SHG members in the Samastipur district took a loan from the SHG to meet the immediate construction expenses. Furthermore, delays in reimbursement of incentive amounts caused hardship to poor households. In Dahod, members kept waiting for months after submitting bills for reimbursement.

Social norms of purity discouraged the idea of using toilets within the residence. It has influenced households to construct toilets outside their dwelling unit. Furthermore, the quality of toilets constructed under public sanitation programmes discourages toilet use. The basic structure of toilets constructed under SBM was often considered substandard by households. Poor quality of doors, roofs, and small pits were the significant causes of not using the toilets in Dahod. They were not confident about the long-term sustainability of twin pit toilets. They feared that twin pit toilets might fill very fast and contaminate groundwater. According to the residents, pits should be ten feet deep instead of only three feet as toilets under SBM were constructed. The households in Bihar and Gujarat preferred septic tanks even if they cost more. Some households opined that the government's incentive amount of Rs. 12000 was too low for the construction of a good-quality toilet. One toilet per household also discouraged toilet use in large families. All the members could not use the toilet at the same time. Hence, they needed to prioritise members' needs for toilet use. Older people had lesser acceptance of behavioural change in sanitation in all the states. They did not find toilets comfortable and believed the

Table 5.3 Percentage Distribution of Households by Reasons for Not Constructing Toilet

	Bihar			*Gujarat*			*Telangana*			*All*
	Sitamarhi	*Samastipur*	*Total*	*Sabarkantha*	*Dahod*	*Total*	*Medak*	*Vikarabad*	*Total*	
Monetary problem	90.00	79.23	82.63	93.75	100.00	98.57	50.00	70.33	68.32	84.45
No benefits	0.00	0.00	0.00	3.13	0.00	0.71	10.00	9.89	9.90	2.55
Lack of proper space	0.00	0.00	0.00	3.13	0.00	0.71	0.00	18.68	16.83	4.18
Do not have own house	10.00	12.31	11.58	0.00	0.00	0.00	0.00	1.10	0.99	5.34
Do not have individual house	0.00	7.69	5.26	0.00	0.00	0.00	0.00	0.00	0.00	2.32
Other reasons/ no particular reason	0.00	0.77	0.53	0.00	0.00	0.00	40.00	0.00	3.96	1.16
Total	100	100	100	100	100	100	100	100	100	100

Source: Primary Survey

Table 5.4 Percentage of Households by Awareness of SBM/Public Sanitation Programme

		Bihar			*Gujarat*			*Telangana*			*All*
		Sitamarhi	*Samastipur*	*Total*	*Sabarkantha*	*Dahod*	*Total*	*Medak*	*Vikarabad*	*Total*	
Awareness of the SBM and/or other sanitation program		69.43	59.91	64.85	71.92	72.82	72.37	92.54	84.08	88.31	74.84
Sources of awareness	Panchayat or political leaders	32.75	29.72	31.29	19.7	13.11	16.38	21.89	0.5	11.19	19.97
	Friends or neighbours	2.62	8.96	5.67	0.49	0	0.24	7.46	1.49	4.48	3.51
	TV or radio	20.96	14.62	17.91	31.53	5.83	18.58	29.35	55.22	42.29	25.96
	Posters	13.54	3.77	8.84	0.49	0	0.24	0.5	0	0.25	3.27
	Social worker or health worker	1.31	6.6	3.85	19.21	54.37	36.92	1.49	0	0.75	13.66
	Social media	0.44	0.94	0.68	18.72	0	9.29	0.5	0	0.25	3.35
	Lecture by national or state-level personalities	0.87	0	0.45	0	0	0	7.46	0	3.73	1.36
	Lecture by local important personalities	0.44	1.42	0.91	0	0	0	22.89	28.86	25.87	8.63

Source: Primary Survey

Table 5.5 Percentage of Households Influenced to Attend Programmes Related to SBM

			Bihar			Gujarat			Telangana			All
			Sitamarhi	Samastipur	Total	Himmatnagar	Dahod	Total	Medak	Vikarabad	Total	
Meeting	Forced/influenced to attend		54.15	74.53	63.95	85.71	88.35	87.04	81.09	94.53	87.81	79.15
	Sources of influence	Panchayat/political leaders	22.27	18.4	20.41	10.34	2.91	6.6	16.42	1.99	9.2	12.3
		Health/social workers	2.62	7.55	4.99	11.82	6.31	9.05	3.98	1	2.49	5.51
		Govt. officials	0	2.83	1.36	0.49	2.43	1.47	10.95	3.98	7.46	3.35
		Friends/neighbours	0	0.47	0.23	0	0	0	2.49	0	1.24	0.48
		Spouse	0	0	0	0	0	0	0	0	0	0
		Other family members	0.44	0.47	0.45	2.46	0.97	1.71	0	0	0	0.72
Song and/or drama function	Forced/influenced to attend		16.59	9.91	13.38	0.99	3.88	2.44	10.45	1.49	5.97	7.43
	Sources of influence	Panchayat/political leaders	14.41	5.66	10.2	0	0.49	0.24	5.97	1	3.48	4.79
		Health/social worker	2.18	3.3	2.72	0.49	0.49	0.49	1.99	0	1	1.44
		Govt. officials	0	0.94	0.45	0	2.43	1.22	6.97	0	3.48	1.68
		Friends/neighbours	0	0	0	0	0.49	0.24	1	0	0.5	0.24
		Spouse	0	0	0	0	0.49	0.24	1	0	0.5	0.24
		Other family members	0	0	0	0.49	0	0.24	0	0	0	0.08

Source: Primary Survey

if political leaders approach them. The role of health and social workers should have been more proactive in this regard. It would have raised consciousness regarding improved sanitation behaviour as a better health practice. There are fewer obligations and more spontaneous participation if health and social workers approach.

In Bihar, community mobilisation and awareness creation for sanitation were conducted through the Bihar Rural Livelihoods Promotion Society, while the district administration was directly involved in implementing SBM(G). Initiatives such as morning vigilance, whistle-blowing, meetings, training, etc. were taken for awareness generation regarding improved sanitation behaviour. In Gujarat, activities undertaken for awareness generation were similar: street play, morning rally, door-to-door visits, training, billboards for SBM, and wall painting. In Telangana, cultural programmes like folk dance were organised for awareness generation. Regular meetings with the SHGs and door-to-door visits were also conducted. In Malkapur village in Medak district, a village-level committee conducted a non-stop sanitation drive for 30 days in the village, where the youth participated enthusiastically.

The attendance of household members in these public programmes was rather slender. The attendance in meetings, awareness and training workshops, or *Melas*[1] was a bit higher with 8% of households attending. Telangana stands out in meetings compared to the other two states (Figure 5.3). Around a quarter of the households had at least one member participating in the meetings. Participation of household members in songs and dramas or display or hoardings and banners was 0.4% and 1%, respectively, taking all the three states together. Despite the initiatives taken by governments for IEC, the community members were not sufficiently aware of the importance of using the toilet, appropriate disposal of faeces, and menstrual hygiene. It was mainly observed in Bihar. Social norms of purity discouraged the idea of using toilets built within a residential dwelling.

Recruitment and appointment of motivators or Swachhagrahis or Swachhata Doots was another critical step to motivate, monitor, and implement the sanitation

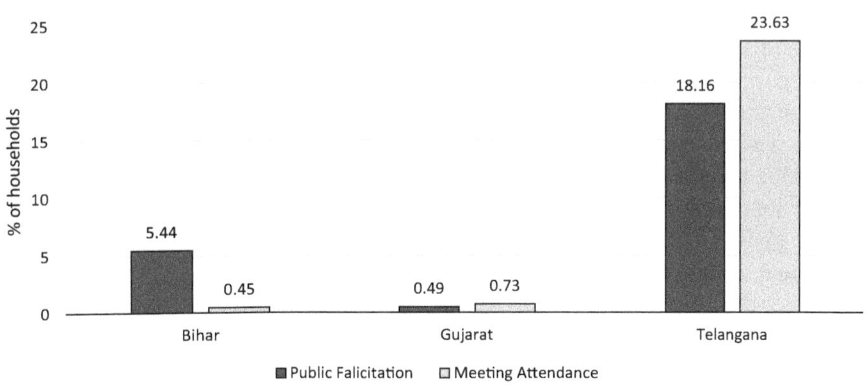

Figure 5.3 Households Felicitated for Contribution in SBM and Attended Meetings.

Source: Primary Survey

programme at the micro level. The state governments appoint them as the key persons for sanitation in Gram Panchayat and a link between Gram Panchayat and the sanitation department of the state government. These motivators were not only present in the SBM structure but also in TSC. Many cadres work in the rural community as Swachhagrahis or Swachhata Doots, but our study reveals that households were largely unaware of them. Overall, 92% of sample households were not aware of them. The laxity on the part of Swachhagrahis to communicate with the rural people could be the reason for the lack of awareness. Generally, staff working in other government programmes such as agriculture or education were given the additional responsibility of SBM. Therefore, they could not provide adequate attention to sanitation work. Our discussions with the villagers revealed that they were aware of the names of the people of the village who were actively working in the sanitation programme. Still, they were not aware of who the Swachhagrahis was.

One crucial strategy for incentivising, boosting morale, and strengthening the campaign is to felicitate citizens for their contribution to SBM. Under the Total Sanitation Campaign, Nirmal Gram Puraskar was launched in 2003 to recognise the efforts of the Panchayats and institutions that have contributed significantly to sanitation coverage. We have enquired whether the households received any felicitation for their contribution towards SBM. Our results reveal that members of 8% of households were felicitated for their contribution to the sanitation programme. However, such facilitation was much more common in Telangana than in Gujarat and Bihar. It may be why 73% of households have a toilet for exclusive use in Telangana, whereas the other two states lag far behind. This achievement was even though 68% of households constructed toilets after the construction of the house. In terms of improved sanitation behaviour, Telangana's people have made better progress than the other two states. Public facilitation may have been necessary for nudging people to adopt better sanitation practices.

Public Health Drive in the Community

The construction and use of the toilet are linked to general cleanliness. Public campaigns and actions regarding cleanliness are likely to have a bearing on adopting improved sanitation behaviour. Most of the villages had abysmal waste management and drainage. Another significant deficit of services commonly observed in villages was the lack of garbage collection. Uncollected garbage is harmful and can subdue the public health benefits of toilet use. In Malkapur village in Medak district, some efforts were made by providing households with two bins for wet and dry garbage. However, these bins were not used by the residents. The drainage system in the village was open, creating mosquitoes and flies. Toilets did not well cover the Wadiyaram village of Medak, but the community spent two hours per day cleaning the village. However, despite efforts to keep the village clean, the drainage condition of the village was poor, and no segregation of household waste took place. There was no arrangement for solid or liquid waste management in the village. In Lingampally village of Vikarabad, communities threw garbage on the road and shared spaces, creating a nuisance of flies and mosquitoes.

Public health campaigns can play an essential role in this regard. These campaigns can nudge villagers and their Panchayats to adopt better public health measures. Our analysis reveals that less than half of the households were aware of drives or campaigns regarding street cleaning, garbage collection, drinking clean water, and health check-ups (Table 5.6). Less than a quarter of households came across campaigns or drives on garbage collection, an essential element of a clean environment. The percentage of households experiencing these public health campaigns or drives was highest in Telangana.

Safe water was an essential issue in Bihar; hence, around one-third of households came across campaigns or drives about drinking clean and safe water. Health check-up drives were observed by more than 80% of households in Dahod and Medak. The high malaria incidence may be the reason for organising health check-up drives in Dahod. The incidence of fever due to diseases other than malaria was also high in Medak, which may have resulted in a higher percentage of households attending the health check-up drives. The discussion on general health and hygiene of sample households has been made in Chapter 4. The lack of garbage cleaning drive in the community may have caused an untidy environment causing the spread of malaria in Dahod. Similarly, a better garbage cleaning drive in the community gave households respite from the mosquito and fly menace in Medak.

Mobile health check-up vans are used to visit the villages in Dahod once a week. These mobile health camps provided essential health consultation and first aid. In case of serious illness, the doctors and nurses of this mobile health van used to refer the patient to the city hospital. The villagers could avail of essential free medication through this health facility. Mobile health van also kept the record of each patient and maintained online data. The main concern of the villagers was that there was no primary health centre in the survey villages. Despite weekly visits by the health check-up vans, medical facilities were inadequate.

Attitude towards Sanitation

Based on existing research and our constant interaction with the target groups, we developed a 20-item instrument measuring the respondents' attitudes towards sanitation. Attitudes are not formed by the utility value of the attitude object but are driven by the combination of utility value and feelings and emotions (Agarwal & Malhotra, 2005). Following Fishbein and Aijen (1975), we used the multi-attribute model of attitude change. These attributes have been analysed separately to understand their variation across regions. Furthermore, we have attempted to identify a handful of broader attitude indicators by clubbing them under broader sub-categories. These broader indicators would indicate the essential factors that determine their attitude and also reveal the factors deemed necessary for forming the attitude towards sanitation.

Understanding individuals' attitudes towards different attributes related to sanitation may help us predict future sanitation behaviour. We have used two techniques to understand this complex issue: one, the Zaltman Metaphor Elicitation

Table 5.6 Percentage Distribution of Households by Experience/Awareness of Public Health Campaigns or Drive

	Bihar			*Gujarat*			*Telangana*			*All*
	Sitamarhi	*Samastipur*	*Total*	*Sabarkantha*	*Dahod*	*Total*	*Medak*	*Vikarabad*	*Total*	
Street cleaning	30.57	16.04	23.58	8.37	58.25	33.5	80.6	20.9	50.75	35.54
Clean water	36.68	26.42	31.75	20.2	5.83	12.96	61.69	20.9	41.29	28.67
Garbage collection	25.33	14.15	19.95	2.46	0	1.22	71.14	23.38	47.26	22.6
Health check-ups	31.88	27.83	29.93	4.93	81.55	43.52	80.6	16.42	48.51	40.34
Total	100	100	100	100	100	100	100	100	100	100

Source: Primary Survey

Technique (ZMET) and two, instruments for measuring different attributes. While ZMET reflects the community's perception about sanitation from their intrinsic thoughts and understanding, measurement of attributes provides the overall perception of community going by indicators set by researchers.

Zaltman Metaphor Elicitation Technique (ZMET)

The Zaltman Metaphor Elicitation Technique (ZMET) enabled us to understand conscious and mainly unconscious thoughts and feelings by exploring people's non-literal or metaphoric expressions. Unconscious and emotional reactions are essential to explore the entire picture of the community's interpretations of motivations (Anca Christina Micu, June 2010). ZMET helps explore the gap between the knowledge about the importance of emotional response in the community's mind. The method taps into the unconscious thoughts and triggers spontaneous and provoked thoughts. ZMET involves symbols to focus on the community's mental models. Thus, ZMET as a tool enabled the exploring and understanding of emotions, preferences, psychological connectedness, and beliefs. This tool is qualitative and time-consuming to be applied using a large sample of participants. One-to-one discussions with households were done to perform the activities of ZMET. We have designed the process to collect and capture five visual images that should represent participants' thoughts and feelings about sanitation and hygiene at the household and community levels. These photographs were mainly clicked by the women or children in the community and facilitated the discussion to contemplate the subconscious thoughts and feelings related to sanitation. ZMET revealed that physical structures, networks, norms, and community beliefs were a few factors influencing the community's perception. Other than this, 50 animated photographs were prepared with the help of training manuals, flip charts, and digital images to provoke the respondent's thoughts on sanitation. The photographs helped the respondents reflect on sanitation beliefs and status at the household and community levels. The responses through ZMET revealed that the emotion of respondents was strongly associated with the initiatives taken for achieving the status of ODF village. The involvement of communities with diverse religions and castes in community events or celebrations provides an immense opportunity for innovation and integration. Respondents broadly compared the programme of the Swachh Bharat Mission with pride, celebration, community mobilisation, and participation. Community perceived personal benefits from toilets. The benefits were perceived to be more to a female for providing dignity, safety, and security. They compared the temples, *Yagya*, and community ceremonies as essential for spiritual or mental well-being.

Similarly, the construction of toilets and usage were essential for physical and social well-being. Some negative emotions were attached to the construction of toilets as it may pollute the groundwater and the sacredness of the house. Positive emotions like pride, ownership, safety, asset creation, and development were directly associated with the villages' construction of toilets and infrastructure.

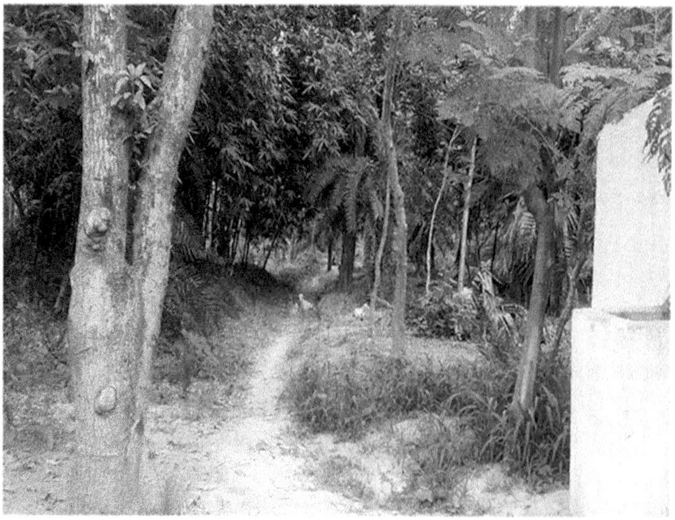

Figure 5.4 Geographical Locations Where the Respondent Lives.
Source: Author – Deepa Gupta

The first picture shows the geographical locations where the respondent lives: the bushes, *kaccha* roads, and no *pucca* houses (Figure 5.4). The household responded that they had made *temporary arrangements to walk. And use the same path when they go for open defecation.*

The household responded, 'We do not have any proper disposal system, so we throw baby faeces here'. This photo depicts where they throw baby faeces and other household waste (Figure 5.5).

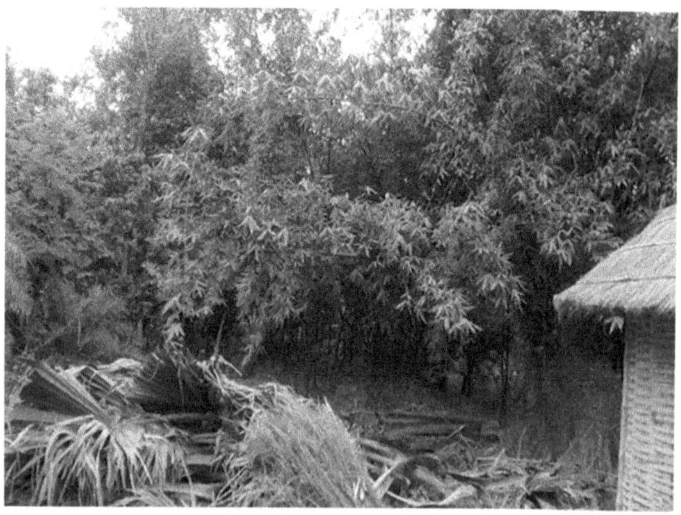

Figure 5.5 Disposal of Baby Faeces.
Source: Author – Deepa Gupta

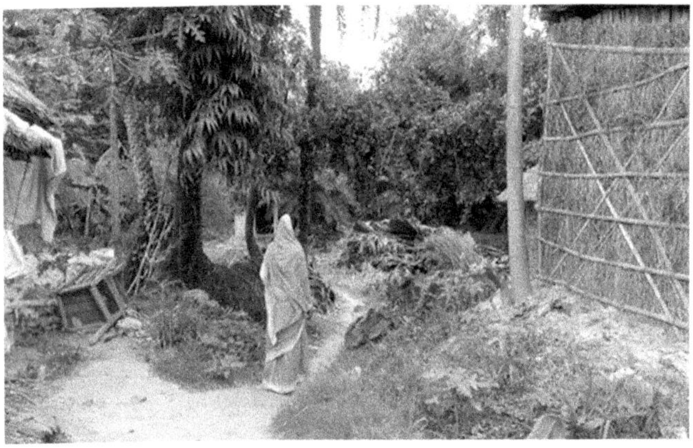

Figure 5.6 Social Norms for Women.

Source: Author – Deepa Gupta

Household responded that 'we are expected to cover our head as it is our culture and tradition (Figure 5.6). Any women who refute to do so will not be considered as good woman. But nobody is bothered that in what conditions we go for defecation. This is us and we go like this every day no matter it's raining or dark'.

Household responded that 'we need temples or any spiritual place for spiritual well-being'. *In a similar way we need toilets and other sanitation facility for physical and personal well*-being (Figure 5.7).

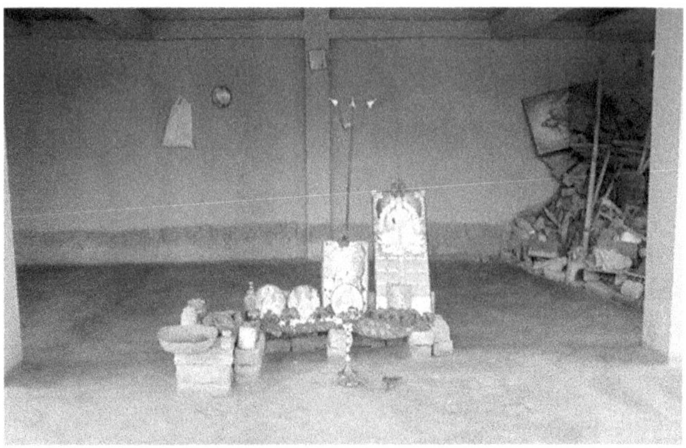

Figure 5.7 Spiritual and Physical Well-Being.

Source: Author – Deepa Gupta

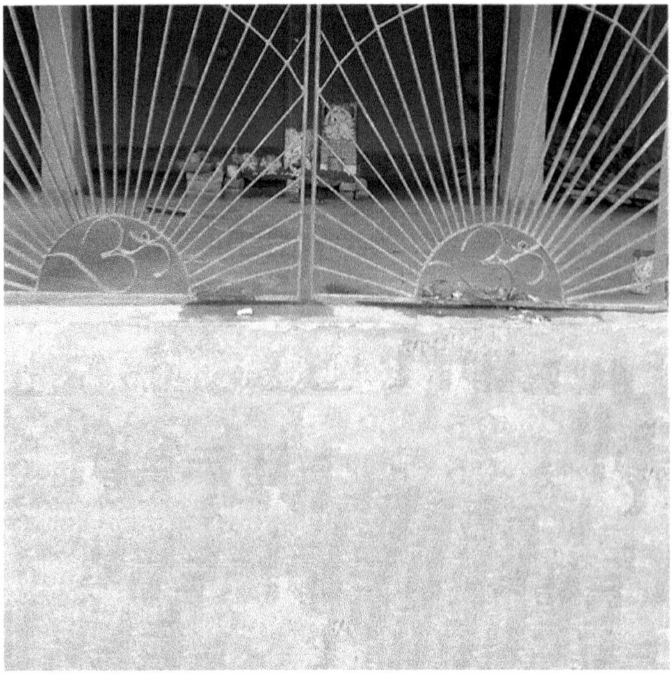

Privacy and safety are essential for women's dignity (Figure 5.8). 'We need the doors in the temple for its safety and security. Similarly, we need toilets with proper doors to have privacy and safety'.

Figure 5.8 Women's Privacy and Safety.
Source: Author – Deepa Gupta

Participants revealed that any event or celebration is not possible without community participation. Likewise, the construction of toilets and their usage could not be possible without community involvement (Figure 5.9).

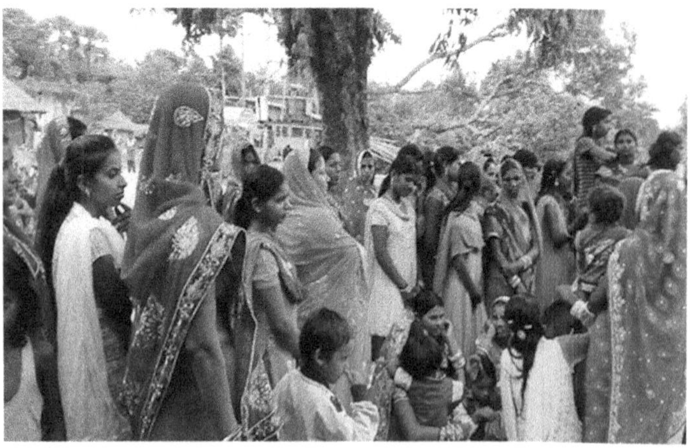

Figure 5.9 Community Participation.
Source: Author – Deepa Gupta

Measurement of Attributes

We had developed a 20-item instrument measuring different attributes regarding sanitation facility, cleanliness, hygiene, and open defecation practices that dominate people's views on sanitation. The respondents were asked to indicate their agreement with the item on a 5-point Likert-type scale: '1' as Completely Disagree, '2' as Disagree, '3' as Indifferent, '4' as Agree, and '5' as Completely Agree. However, most responses gravitated towards mid ranges (between 2 and 4); the extremes (1 and 5) were almost absent. We clubbed the outliers 'Completely Disagree' (1) with Disagree (2) and 'Completely Agree' (5) with 'Agree' (4) and thus retained the three points 'Agree', 'Indifferent', and 'Disagree'. The statements were intended to measure the respondent's positive attitude towards sanitation. We included ten positively and ten negatively worded items to avoid acquiescence bias. We have subdivided the attitudes towards sanitation into a few sub-categories: Shame, Safety, and Convenience; Community Health and Hygiene; Necessity or Priority; and Quality of Infrastructure.

Shame, Safety, and Convenience

Most survey villages consider open defecation unsafe for women and everybody. The majority considered open defecation shameful for women (Table 5.7). Nevertheless, only around 60% of respondents believe that open defecation provides no privacy. More surprisingly, 42% in Telangana and 31% in Bihar disagree that open defecation provides no privacy. Taken both the statements together, one may infer that although people considered open defecation shameful for women, they did not consider open defecation negatively affecting women's privacy. The seemingly contradictory thinking may be explained by past research that privacy concern is much less critical to Indians than their American cohorts (Malhotra et al., 2004). Similarly, in the Indian context, women have a special obligation to protect themselves from 'shame' by observing certain cultural and social norms (Qamar, 2015) because social norms play an essential role where women's movement outside the home is restricted.

Around one-fourth of respondents in Sabarkantha disagreed with the idea that open defecation provides no privacy. Moreover, one-fourth of respondents agreed with the idea that open defecation provides an opportunity to discuss important matters with friends. Overall, in Sabarkantha, open defecation was not viewed negatively. This observation is surprising as 72% of the respondents are aware of SBM or any other government sanitation programme. One plausible reason behind it could be that household heads are more aged in Sabarkantha compared to other districts. In Sabarkantha, around one-fourth of household heads were aged 60 years or older, while the same holds for 15% of households in the overall sample (see Chapter 4). Older people may be less averse to open defecation.

Community Health and Hygiene

The community's perception of the harmful effects of open defecation has been analysed through questions interrogating their opinion on it. Three-fourths of the

Table 5.7 Percentage Distribution of Households by Shame, Safety, and Convenience Attitudes

Attitude	*Opinion*	*Bihar*			*Gujarat*			*Telangana*			*All*
		Sitamarhi	*Samastipur*	*Total*	*Sabarkantha*	*Dahod*	*Total*	*Medak*	*Vikarabad*	*Total*	
Open defecation is unsafe for women	Disagree	0.44	0.94	0.68	3.45	0.49	1.96	0.5	3.48	1.99	1.52
	Indifferent	0.44	0	0.23	6.9	1.46	4.16	0	2.99	1.49	1.92
	Agree	99.13	99.06	99.09	89.66	98.06	93.89	99.5	93.53	96.52	96.57
	Total	100	100	100	100	100	100	100	100	100	100
Open defecation during night is unsafe for everybody	Disagree	1.31	3.3	2.27	6.9	3.88	5.38	1.49	4.98	3.23	3.59
	Indifferent	1.75	7.55	4.54	8.37	3.4	5.87	0	1.99	1	3.83
	Agree	96.94	89.15	93.2	84.73	92.72	88.75	98.51	93.03	95.77	92.57
	Total	100	100	100	100	100	100	100	100	100	100
Open defecation is shameful for women	Disagree	0.44	0.94	0.68	2.46	0.97	1.71	1	3.48	2.24	1.52
	Indifferent	0	0	0	8.87	0.97	4.89	0	1.99	1	1.92
	Agree	99.56	99.06	99.32	88.67	98.06	93.4	99	94.53	96.77	96.57
	Total	100	100	100	100	100	100	100	100	100	100
Open defecation provides no privacy	Disagree	33.62	27.83	30.84	23.65	10.19	16.87	41.79	42.29	42.04	29.87
	Indifferent	0.44	0.47	0.45	15.27	6.31	10.76	8.46	25.87	17.16	9.19
	Agree	65.94	71.7	68.71	61.08	83.5	72.37	49.75	31.84	40.8	60.94
	Total	100	100	100	100	100	100	100	100	100	100
During open defecation people discuss important things with friends	Disagree	58.95	60.85	59.86	56.16	31.55	43.77	71.14	34.83	52.99	52.4
	Indifferent	37.55	21.7	29.93	18.23	62.14	40.34	14.43	47.76	31.09	33.71
	Agree	3.49	17.45	10.2	25.62	6.31	15.89	14.43	17.41	15.92	13.9
	Total	100	100	100	100	100	100	100	100	100	100

Source: Primary Survey

respondents disagreed with the idea that open defecation does not have any harmful effect (Table 5.8). Furthermore, 72% of respondents opined that open defecation causes diarrhoea. The realisation of the ill effects of open defecation on health seems to be highest in the Dahod district. It may be due to the higher consciousness of people on public health due to the high incidence of fever, including malaria, in the district, as discussed in Chapter 4.

We have enquired about the general cleanliness of the villages. It was observed that a little less than half of the respondents believed that their village was clean and disagreed that the sanitation condition in their village was very bad. In this respect, Gujarat is better than the other two states, while Bihar is at the bottom. The cleanliness of the villages has a bearing on the nuisance of mosquitoes and flies.

Priority of Sanitation

We have enquired about the priority of toilets by juxtaposing the importance of different goods, amenities, and infrastructure per respondents' opinions. Cellular communication is one of the essential means of information, especially for livelihood opportunities for rural households. Moreover, due to increasing migration, cellular communication is essential to keep track of household issues by the migrants. Despite the significance of mobile phones, 85% of respondents did not find mobile phones more important than the toilet (Table 5.9). Another critical and cheap mode of communication for rural India, the bicycle, was found to be less critical than toilets by 86% of respondents. However, regarding the road, it was observed that only 20% of respondents agreed that roads were more critical than sanitation, while 62% of households disagreed. It implies that according to a household's preference, sanitation ranked below the basic public infrastructure like a road but ranked above of personal necessities like mobile phones and bicycles.

There are variations in the household's priorities. In Samastipur and Sabarkantha, more than 10% of respondents felt that mobile phones and bicycles are more important than toilets. A higher percentage of respondents from both the survey districts in Bihar considers that roads are more important than toilets. A considerable percentage of households in the Sabarkantha district of Gujarat responded similarly. A higher proportion of respondents with a regular wage or salary earnings in Bihar compared to the other states (as discussed in Chapter 4) could be one of the primary reasons for the importance of roads in Bihar. People require better road infrastructure for commuting. As around one-fourth of the respondent household heads were aged 60 years or more in Sabarkantha, which is higher than in other districts, their priority of toilets is much less than other necessities and infrastructure. Overall, the results imply that developing basic public infrastructure and communication is essential.

The priority of behaviour change may also depend on the prevalence of open defecation in the area. The higher the prevalence of open defecation, the greater the possibility of people sticking to their old habits of open defecation. Dependence of individual actions on others' behaviour has been conceptualised by Bicchieri (2016) as empirical expectations which influence collective behaviour, such as open defecation. Our survey results suggest that more than one-third of the respondents

Table 5.8 Percentage Distribution of Households by Community Health and Hygiene Attitudes

Attitude	*Opinion*	*Bihar*			*Gujarat*			*Telangana*			*All*
		Sitamarhi	*Samastipur*	*Total*	*Sabarkantha*	*Dahod*	*Total*	*Medak*	*Vikarabad*	*Total*	
Open defecation causes no harm	Disagree	55.02	75.94	65.08	64.04	91.75	78	78.61	85.57	82.09	74.76
	Indifferent	2.18	7.08	4.54	14.29	5.34	9.78	8.46	9.95	9.2	7.75
	Agree	42.79	16.98	30.39	21.67	2.91	12.22	12.94	4.48	8.71	17.49
	Total	100	100	100	100	100	100	100	100	100	100
Open defecation is a cause of diarrhoea	Disagree	57.64	31.6	45.12	8.37	10.68	9.54	7.96	7.96	7.96	21.57
	Indifferent	3.49	1.42	2.49	14.29	14.56	14.43	2.99	3.48	3.23	6.63
	Agree	38.86	66.98	52.38	77.34	74.76	76.04	89.05	88.56	88.81	71.81
	Total	100	100	100	100	100	100	100	100	100	100
My village is very clean	Disagree	75.11	58.96	67.35	14.85	7.28	11.03	28.86	91.54	60.2	46.68
	Indifferent	3.93	2.83	3.4	8.91	16.99	12.99	1.99	1.49	1.74	6
	Agree	20.96	38.21	29.25	76.24	75.73	75.98	69.15	6.97	38.06	47.32
	Total	100	100	100	100	100	100	100	100	100	100
Sanitation condition in my village is very bad	Disagree	24.89	33.49	29.02	49.75	73.79	61.86	72.14	46.77	59.45	49.52
	Indifferent	14.85	10.85	12.93	20.2	15.53	17.85	4.98	0.5	2.74	11.26
	Agree	60.26	55.66	58.05	30.05	10.68	20.29	22.89	52.74	37.81	39.22
	Total	100	100	100	100	100	100	100	100	100	100

Source: Own Primary Survey, 2018

Table 5.9 Percentage Distribution of Households by Priority of Sanitation

Attitude	*Opinion*	*Bihar*			*Gujarat*			*Telangana*			*All*
		Sitamarhi	*Samastipur*	*Total*	*Sabarkantha*	*Dahod*	*Total*	*Medak*	*Vikarabad*	*Total*	
Mobile phone is more necessary than a toilet	Disagree	83.84	81.13	82.54	76.35	90.78	83.62	91.54	87.06	89.3	85.06
	Indifferent	13.1	5.19	9.3	12.32	4.85	8.56	6.47	8.96	7.71	8.55
	Agree	3.06	13.68	8.16	11.33	4.37	7.82	1.99	3.98	2.99	6.39
	Total	100	100	100	100	100	100	100	100	100	100
Here, bicycle is more important than a toilet	Disagree	83.41	83.02	83.22	77.34	90.29	83.86	92.04	91.54	91.79	86.18
	Indifferent	7.42	5.19	6.35	11.82	6.8	9.29	6.97	6.97	6.97	7.51
	Agree	9.17	11.79	10.43	10.84	2.91	6.85	1	1.49	1.24	6.31
	Total	100	100	100	100	100	100	100	100	100	100
Roads are more important than sanitation in the village	Disagree	61.57	62.74	62.13	59.61	28.64	44.01	73.13	88.56	80.85	62.22
	Indifferent	1.31	3.77	2.49	18.23	59.22	38.88	15.42	8.46	11.94	17.41
	Agree	37.12	33.49	35.37	22.17	12.14	17.11	11.44	2.99	7.21	20.37
	Total	100	100	100	100	100	100	100	100	100	100
Open defecation is normal practice here	Disagree	35.81	24.06	30.16	47.29	79.61	63.57	69.65	45.77	57.71	49.92
	Indifferent	14.85	9.43	12.24	28.57	10.68	19.56	10.95	1.99	6.47	12.78
	Agree	49.34	66.51	57.6	24.14	9.71	16.87	19.4	52.24	35.82	37.3

Source: Own Primary Survey, 2018

believed that open defecation was a regular practice in their area. It is a significant hindrance to spreading improved sanitation behaviour.

The Pleasure of Open Defecation

Open defecation is often an age-old practice. People may have developed a habit of open defecation and are unwilling to leave the old practice. They may be deriving utility and pleasure out of open defecation. People may develop and strengthen their social network during their journey for open defecation. These networks may be vital in resolving their life and livelihood problems. Furthermore, people may find it challenging to use the toilet.

A substantial proportion of the respondents opined that there are benefits of open defecation as, during open defecation, important matters can be discussed with friends (Table 5.10). Although around half of the respondents disagreed with such benefits of open defecation, around one-third were indifferent about it. The latter indicates that developing a social network during open defecation was somewhat crucial for the villagers. Within the districts, Sabarkantha had the highest proportion of respondents who agreed. More old-aged household heads could be the reason behind such a preference for open defecation. For 17% of the respondents, open defecation was used for enjoying fresh air (Table 5.10). The preference, for this reason, was highest in Vikarabad, where 46% of respondents showed such preference. Vikarabad district had the highest percentage (87%) of households having a primary occupation as self-employed in agriculture. Due to access to agricultural fields and open spaces, they might be more inclined to seek fresh air.

Toilet Infrastructure

The affordability and comfort of using a toilet have been examined to understand households' attitudes towards toilet infrastructure. Flush or pour toilets were not costly for 48% of the households, while around one-third were indifferent (Table 5.11). A higher proportion of households in Bihar considers the toilets very costly. It could be due to their worse economic condition, as explained in Chapter 4.

The space within the toilets is small and can make it uncomfortable for people to use if they are not used to a closed space for defecation. More than half of the households did not find that toilets were closed and so challenging to use, but around 21% thought so (Table 5.11). Interestingly, such opinion among respondents was highest in Gujarat. It may be due to the higher aspiration level of the region's people. The per capita expenses in Sabarkantha were the highest among the survey districts (see Chapter 4). Dahod is a district with a large tribal population and forest land. Hence, people of the district may find closed spaces like toilets uncomfortable.

Hygiene of Flush/Pour Toilets

Households' perception of the toilets' hygiene and ease of maintenance has a lot of bearing on their use. If households find it hygienic and safe, they are more likely to

Table 5.10 Percentage Distribution of Households by Their Opinion on Pleasure of Open Defecation

Attitude	*Opinion*	*Bihar*			*Gujarat*			*Telangana*			*All*
		Sitamarhi	*Samastipur*	*Total*	*Sabarkantha*	*Dahod*	*Total*	*Medak*	*Vikarabad*	*Total*	
During open defecation we discuss important things with friends	Disagree	58.95	60.85	59.86	56.16	31.55	43.77	71.14	34.83	52.99	52.4
	Indifferent	37.55	21.7	29.93	18.23	62.14	40.34	14.43	47.76	31.09	33.71
	Agree	3.49	17.45	10.2	25.62	6.31	15.89	14.43	17.41	15.92	13.9
	Total	100	100	100	100	100	100	100	100	100	100
Open defecation is pleasant because of open air	Disagree	69.87	71.23	70.52	59.61	83.98	71.88	74.63	35.32	54.98	65.97
	Indifferent	26.2	15.09	20.86	20.69	7.77	14.18	14.93	18.41	16.67	17.33
	Agree	3.93	13.68	8.62	19.7	8.25	13.94	10.45	46.27	28.36	16.69
	Total	100	100	100	100	100	100	100	100	100	100

Source: Own Primary Survey, 2018

Table 5.11 Percentage Distribution of Households by Their Opinion on Toilet Infrastructure

		Bihar			*Gujarat*			*Telangana*			*All*
		Sitamarhi	*Samastipur*	*Total*	*Sabarkantha*	*Dahod*	*Total*	*Medak*	*Vikarabad*	*Total*	
Flush/pour toilet is very costly	Disagree	36.68	50.47	43.31	56.65	17.48	36.92	71.64	55.72	63.68	47.76
	Indifferent	27.95	17.45	22.9	31.03	72.82	52.08	24.88	36.32	30.6	34.9
	Agree	35.37	32.08	33.79	12.32	9.71	11	3.48	7.96	5.72	17.33
	Total	100	100	100	100	100	100	100	100	100	100
Toilets are closed, so I am unable to breathe	Disagree	79.04	76.42	77.78	21.67	26.7	24.21	72.64	65.17	68.91	57.43
	Indifferent	19.65	16.04	17.91	26.6	21.36	23.96	22.39	25.37	23.88	21.81
	Agree	1.31	7.55	4.31	51.72	51.94	51.83	4.98	9.45	7.21	20.77
	Total	100	100	100	100	100	100	100	100	100	100

Source: Primary Survey

use toilets. If households find it difficult to maintain, they are less likely to use it. Social norms about sanitation behaviour may also play an essential role in households' perceptions regarding the use of the toilet. The matter of concern was that half of the respondents felt that toilets were not safe to use (Table 5.12). This perception was highest in Gujarat and lowest in Bihar. Possible contamination of groundwater may be one of the reasons for considering toilet use unsafe. A substantial proportion of the respondents believed toilets were difficult to maintain, although more than half disagreed. Again, a higher proportion of respondents from Sabarkantha felt that toilets were difficult to maintain than respondents of any other district.

The construction of toilets inside a home would provide better access to a toilet. It is likely to have better use of a toilet. Our survey results reveal that 11% of households felt that toilets inside the home are unhygienic. However, 63% of households disagree with the opinion. The poor quality of infrastructure may be one reason for such an opinion. The other reason could be entrenched social norms of purity. Himmantnagar district again stands out where more than one-fourth of the respondents feel that the toilet inside the home was unhygienic.

There may have been a genuine reason for considering the toilet inside a home as hygienic. If the toilet gives a bad smell, households may consider using it unhygienic inside the home. In this case, around 9% agreed with the opinion. Interestingly, almost a similar percentage of respondents in Samastipur and Sabarkantha felt that toilets emitted a bad smell. Still, a much higher proportion of respondents in Sabarkantha opined that the toilet inside the home was unhygienic. It implies that social norms of purity were more entrenched in Sabarkantha.

Results of Factor Analysis

Factor analysis is a common technique used in psychology and social sciences to identify any hidden essential variables as a combination of different observed variables (Crawford & Lomas, 1980; Line, 1994). It is a data reduction technique that identifies an underlying relationship from a set of variables. Thus, different sets of variables represent different underlying variables. The variables are combined using objectively determined weight, called factor loadings. In this process of combining variables, the smallest number of independent summary variables are created and interpreted to meet the research needs.

Before factor analysis, all the negatively worded items were reverse coded so that all items were in the same direction. We wanted to know the extent to which the respondents had a positive attitude towards sanitation, i.e., whether open defecation is shameful for women or open defecation is the cause of diarrhoea. The factor analysis revealed that two items or variables did not result in any significant factors and two items had almost equal loadings on two factors. These four items were dropped. We conducted factor analysis using the varimax rotation method with 16 items, resulting in five significant factors – Shame and Safety, Community health and hygiene, Structural barrier, Sanitation Environment, and Household priority. These factors explain 64.26% of the total variance. The mean, standard deviations, factor loadings of all items, and variance explained are presented in Table 5.13.

Table 5.12 Percentage Distribution of Households by Hygiene and Safety of Toilets

Attitude	*Opinion*	*Bihar*			*Gujarat*			*Telangana*			*All*
		Sitamarhi	*Samastipur*	*Total*	*Sabarkantha*	*Dahod*	*Total*	*Medak*	*Vikarabad*	*Total*	
Toilet safe to use	Disagree	35.81	24.06	30.16	47.29	79.61	63.57	69.65	45.77	57.71	49.92
	Indifferent	14.85	9.43	12.24	28.57	10.68	19.56	10.95	1.99	6.47	12.78
	Agree	49.34	66.51	57.6	24.14	9.71	16.87	19.4	52.24	35.82	37.3
	Total	100	100	100	100	100	100	100	100	100	100
Toilet difficult to maintain	Disagree	82.53	71.7	77.32	30.54	17.96	24.21	75.12	60.2	67.66	56.87
	Indifferent	14.41	21.23	17.69	29.56	71.84	50.86	13.93	30.35	22.14	29.95
	Agree	3.06	7.08	4.99	39.9	10.19	24.94	10.95	9.45	10.2	13.18
	Total	100	100	100	100	100	100	100	100	100	100
The toilet inside a home is unclean	Disagree	88.65	81.13	85.03	47.29	21.84	34.47	80.1	57.71	68.91	63.34
	Indifferent	8.73	7.55	8.16	26.11	68.93	47.68	11.44	36.32	23.88	26.12
	Agree	2.62	11.32	6.8	26.6	9.22	17.85	8.46	5.97	7.21	10.54
	Total	100	100	100	100	100	100	100	100	100	100
Toilet gives very bad smell	Disagree	75.98	71.23	73.7	59.11	11.17	34.96	63.68	56.72	60.2	56.71
	Indifferent	19.65	13.68	16.78	29.56	79.13	54.52	22.39	41.79	32.09	34.03
	Agree	4.37	15.09	9.52	11.33	9.71	10.51	13.93	1.49	7.71	9.27
	Total	100	100	100	100	100	100	100	100	100	100

Source: Primary Survey

Table 5.13 Factor Loadings for Perception and Attitude towards Sanitation

Component Factor			*1*	*2*	*3*	*4*	*5*
Items for Attitude towards Sanitation	*Mean*	*SD*	*Shame and Safety*	*Community Health and Hygiene*	*Structural Barrier*	*Sanitation Environment*	*Household Priority*
Total variance explained (cumulative %)			20.693	36.117	46.992	56.590	64.258
Open defecation is unsafe for women	4.55	0.625	0.908				
Open defecation is shameful for women	4.54	0.626	0.882				
Open defecation during night is unsafe for everybody	4.46	0.767	0.799				
Roads are more important than sanitation in the village (r)	3.44	1.181		0.797			
Open defecation causes no harm (r)	3.68	1.184		0.736			
Open defecation is a cause of diarrhoea	3.65	1.275		0.520			
Flush/pour toilet gives very bad smell (r)	3.74	1.007			0.827		
Flush/pour toilet inside home is unhygienic (r)	3.85	1.057			0.792		
Flush/pour toilet is very costly (r)	3.47	1.092			0.630		
My village is very clean	3.06	1.346				0.814	
Flush/pour toilets are closed, so I am unable to breathe (r)	2.45	1.168				0.644	
Open defecation is normal practice here (r)	3.19	1.082				0.532	
Open defecation provides no privacy	3.45	1.274				0.458	
Mobile phone is more necessary than a toilet (r)	4.11	0.882					0.836
Here, bicycle is more than a toilet (r)	4.15	0.879					0.720
Open defecation is pleasant because of open air (r)	3.60	1.101					0.667

Note: Items marked as (r) are reverse coded

Factor 1 (shame and safety) had the highest variance explained (20.69%), with three items loaded with very high factor loadings. One of the items was 'Open defecation is unsafe for women'. While women move out of their homes for open defecation, they become visible to others and get exposed to other hazards like harm caused by men or other miscreants. They are visible for open defecation; women lose privacy which is shameful to them. To avoid loss of privacy, women may choose to go out for defecation when only a few are present outside, which exposes them to different threats challenging their safety and security. To avoid shame, many women in rural areas go out for open defecation early in the morning, before sunrise and in the evening when it is dark. However, going out in the dark is also unsafe for many of them.

Factor 2 (community health and hygiene) explained 15.42% of the variance. It had three items which tried to capture the respondents' beliefs regarding the health and hygiene consequences of open defecation. There were two negatively coded items, and one was a positively coded item (open defecation is a cause of diarrhoea). The responses establish that community health and hygiene is also an essential factor in the minds of the respondents. However, in terms of precedence, it is lower than the shame and safety dimension.

Factor 3 (structural barrier) represents problems caused by the poor quality of structure of the toilet. Poor quality may lead to bad smell, unhygienic, and costly to construct and maintain. It explained 10.87% of the total variance. The structural barriers considered are physical discomfort and non-acceptance of the structure of the toilet in the household. It is a significant barrier that prevents many individuals from using the toilet. Factor 4 (sanitation environment) such as sanitation environment and affordability have a significant role in influencing people's views on sanitation, similar to social norms (e.g. open defecation is standard practice here). The factor explained 9.6% of the total variance. Factor 5 (household priority) is about the household's priorities over durable goods, and pleasure vis-à-vis sanitation are critical factors. The factor explained 7.69% of the total variance.

Overall, the results imply that privacy, safety, and security, especially for the womenfolk, are most important in shaping people's attitudes towards sanitation. Health and hygiene considerations are the second most crucial factor in people's perception of improved sanitation behaviour. Structural barriers include infrastructure cost and quality and people's sense of purity, which is the third most important factor contributing to people's attitude towards sanitation. The financial ability of the household has a lot of bearing on structural barriers. It is interesting to note that economic difficulties weigh much lesser than safety and security. Perception of hygiene of toilet use inside the house may also be determined by structural factors like social norms.

Factors that emerge as less necessary in forming attributes towards sanitation are sanitation environment and household priorities. The cleanliness of the village, comfort in using the toilet, the prevalence of open defecation in the village, and privacy issues are essential components of the sanitation environment. The lesser importance of sanitation environment in attitude towards sanitation implies that sanitation attitude is majorly a private affair. Social practices and norms may have bearings on it but only mildly. Individual preferences for toilet use are mainly attributable to safety, security, and public health concerns. Other competition needs of individuals such as electronic gadgets or pleasure of open defecation are ranked much lower in the order.

What We Learnt?

This chapter attempted to analyse the priority of the households for toilet construction, reasons for constructing and not constructing a toilet, awareness about public sanitation programmes, public health drive in the community, and attitude towards sanitation. Overall, the priority of toilet construction is less for the survey households as understood from the time of construction of the toilet. Only 14% constructed toilets at the time of house construction, while 53% of households constructed them later.

Convenience and privacy were the two most important reasons for toilet construction. While privacy was the primary concern in Bihar, convenience was the major reason for toilet construction in Gujarat. Moreover, potential health benefits were also one of the significant reasons for toilet construction in Bihar. One of the minor reasons for toilet construction is a significant concern, force, and coercion by officials or leaders. It was mainly observed in Telangana, especially in Medak. The pressure of influential individuals should be avoided in implementing government programmes. The influence for toilet construction was majorly self and spouse. Financial constraint was one of the primary reasons for not constructing a toilet. Constructing toilets within residential dwellings was discouraged due to social norms of purity. More than 95% of households were willing to construct a toilet in the future, but a concrete plan is generally absent.

The awareness of the public sanitation programme, Swachh Bharat Mission (SBM), was high in the survey villages. One-fourth of the households were made aware through TV or radio broadcastings. The awareness was also spread through meetings and public functions like songs and drama. Most households that attended meetings were influenced or forced, while a much less percentage of people attended public functions through influence and force. It implies that more public functions should be organised to motivate people to attend IEC programmes spontaneously.

Looking into the people's understanding, emotions, and attitudes towards sanitation, we observe that social norms hindered the use of the toilet. However, there was a demand for toilet construction with doors and other safety measures, especially from women. They considered community participation essential for an overall change in sanitation behaviour. Our analysis reveals that knowing about SBM does not change people's attitudes against open defecation. A substantial proportion of households believed that open defecation does not threaten privacy.

Similarly, a substantial proportion believed that open defecation provided them pleasure and an opportunity to discuss important matters. There were revealed attitudes towards the toilet as well. More than 80% of respondents believed that mobile phones and bicycles are less important than the toilet. Almost half of the respondents did not find flush or pour-flush toilets costly. More than half of the respondents did not find difficulty in closed and small space within toilets. The analysis of attitudes towards sanitation further reveals that fear of possible contamination of groundwater due to the use of twin pit toilets was palpable. Households felt that it was challenging to maintain a toilet, and it was unhygienic to use the toilet inside the home. The analysis confirms that privacy, safety, and security influence people's attitudes towards sanitation. Economic ability matters in people's attitude towards sanitation but to a lesser extent than privacy and safety. Health and hygiene concerns and a sense of purity affect people's attitudes towards sanitation differently.

Note

1 Melas are village fairs.

6 Household Characteristics and Sanitation

Sanitation is a quasi-public good as it is one of our most private behaviours with some of our most public impacts (McGranahan, 2015). Due to the externality in sanitation services, individual health benefits of toilet construction may not be realised only through a modest increase in household toilets and even a modest reduction of open defecation (Patil et al., 2014). The private demands do not consider the social benefit; therefore, commercial enterprises are not motivated enough to produce sufficient sanitation to satisfy social benefit (McGranahan, 2015). Hence, market intervention is required to produce sanitation up to the optimal level. Public sanitation programmes in Asia and Africa are testimony to this reality. However, despite prolonged efforts, globally, 3.6 billion people lack access to safely managed sanitation services.[1] The deficiency may be due to a lack of effort by the government. However, as sanitation behaviour is intricately driven by private choice, household characteristics, including demography and socio-economic conditions, matter greatly. In addition, households may also be influenced by government policies such as subsidies and information, education, and communication (IEC).

Along with household demographics, the norms regarding human waste vary across cultures and ethnic identities (Jewitt, 2011). In 'feacophobic' (Buit & Jansen, 2016, p. 97) cultures, handling of shit is well accepted, but in feacophobic cultures handling shit or words that describe it is considered abhorring, ritually polluting, and offensive (Esrey et al., 1998; van der Geest, 1998). In India, handling of human waste is culturally denigrated by Hindus and is considered to be the work of backward castes or untouchables (Ramaswamy, 2005). De (2018) observed that Hindus and backward castes are more likely to practice open defecation or not use the toilet. Furthermore, social networks about sanitation profoundly impact access and attitudes towards toilets (De et al., 2021). However, such cultural relegation of handling waste is not observed in Asian countries like China and Vietnam (Esrey et al., 1998; Hart-Davis, 2008). Hence, it is essential to examine whether household sanitation behaviour is influenced by the cultural and ethnic identity of the households.

The unavailability of basic infrastructures like bathrooms and toilets will likely negatively impact household sanitation. It is because they are complementary services and improve life leading to aspiration for a better life. De (2018) observed that access to water supply and bathroom impact access to toilet and its use. The income of households also plays a significant role in toilet access. Along with basic

DOI: 10.4324/9781032726267-6

infrastructure and income, other public actions and the external environment will likely influence household sanitation decisions. According to O'Reilly and Louis (2014), long-term multi-scalar political will, including that of government and NGOs, and political ecology, including access to water and land use, has a bearing on sanitation behaviour. Social pressure, including person-to-person contact, is also considered an essential factor. All together, these three factors constitute a toilet tripod.

In this chapter, we analyse the determinants of access to toilets and their use. We have examined the relationship between sanitation behaviour and different socio-economic factors. Concerning sanitation behaviour, we have considered toilet access and use. Different socio-economic factors considered are ethnic identity and the economic condition of households. Access to household and social infrastructures like water supply and bathroom are considered to understand how they impact toilet access and use. The cost of toilet construction may emerge as a constraining factor. Hence, we have discussed the cost of toilet construction and the subsidy provided by the government to cover the construction cost. The subsidy provided by the government through the public sanitation programme also reveals the government's political will to usher in behaviour change in sanitation.

Drivers of Toilet Use

The construction and use of a toilet by a person are driven by a complex set of socio-economic and institutional factors. These factors affect toilet construction and use directly as well as indirectly. The earlier studies have attempted to determine the factors that determine sanitation behaviour (see De, 2018; De et al., 2021) but it requires a holistic understanding and clarity of thought on the primary drivers of behavioural change. The latter would help in public action for total sanitation. The household's economic condition could be one of the significant reasons for toilet construction. Government subsidies provided through public sanitation programmes may be helpful in this context. However, with an increase in government spending on sanitation, the use of toilets may not automatically rise (De, 2018; Coffey & Spears, 2017). Several factors, including caste and attitudes, may hinder efforts to improve toilet use. The use of the toilet may also depend on access to the basic infrastructure of the household. The household's economic condition may also determine basic infrastructures and services, which can have a bearing on toilet use.

There are two types of infrastructure accessed by the household: social infrastructure and household infrastructure. One of the critical social infrastructures that might have a bearing on toilet use is access to water supply for drinking, washing, and cleaning. If water sources are far or the water supply is inadequate for drinking or other activities, it would create water stress. Households would not be willing to use the toilet under water stress if there was an option for open defecation. A critical household infrastructure is a bathroom. Bathrooms are more frequently used during the day than the toilet. Hence, the household may rank the bathroom more critical than the toilet. If the household does not have a bathroom as well as structures were inappropriate for them. They found it challenging to give up their old practices of open defecation.

Along with older people, children and adults in Telangana were found to be reluctant to use the toilet as they were unwilling to change their sanitation behaviour. People felt that toilets were filthy with a foul smell. They felt claustrophobic within toilets. Some children became more reluctant to use the toilet when the habit of using the toilet was not developed in primary school or *Anganwadis*. The children often found toilets in primary school or *Anganwadis* unclean or closed.

Public Awareness

The major sanitation programme rolled over during the survey was the Swachh Bharat Mission (SBM). Our survey reveals that three-fourths of the survey households were aware of SBM (Table 5.4). This awareness was highest in Telangana and lowest in Bihar. The medium of information was primarily broadcast media like television and radio. One-fourth of the households received information about SBM through television and radio. In Gujarat, households knew about SBM through a campaign 'Swachhata Hi Sewa' broadcast through television. Another essential medium of awareness generation was social media, mainly observed in the Dahod district and, to a large extent, in Sabarkantha.

On the other hand, Panchayat or local political leaders were the significant facilitators of information on SBM, especially in Bihar. Awareness generation through lectures delivered by nationally or locally influential personalities had a moderate impact on awareness of SBM. It implies that awareness about public sanitation programmes is best generated through popular media and one-to-one interactions.

The awareness regarding public sanitation programmes such as SBM is spread through meetings and public functions like songs and drama, which sensitise people through entertainment. The government and non-government organisations were taking many initiatives to promote sanitation behaviour among individuals, households, and communities. Campaigns, rallies, workshops, 'Nukkad Natak' (street plays), songs, plays, and IEC material were some of the initiatives of the government, NGOs and CSR groups for awareness creation. We have attempted to understand whether any household member was influenced or forced to attend these programmes. Our results reveal that around 80% of households were influenced or forced to attend the meeting, and 7% of households were influenced to attend public functions. The popularity of these latter programmes might have driven the extent of influencing the population. While fewer households were influenced to attend meetings in Bihar compared to the other two states, a higher percentage of households in Bihar was influenced to attend entertainment programmes like songs and drama (Table 5.5). Hence, the IEC instrument varies across regions.

In both meetings and entertainment programmes were Panchayat or political leaders, followed by health or social workers (Table 5.5). It was true in Bihar and Telangana, but in Gujarat, the social and health workers play a more critical role. The influence of political leaders and institutions is understood from public actions for IEC. However, there are chances that people feel obliged to attend these programmes a toilet, then the bathroom would need to be constructed first. Having and using a bathroom is an initial stage of uplifting living standards; toilet construction and use would happen later. The attitude towards toilet use may be highly influenced by caste, religion, or other social identities. The social identity of the household is linked to social norms, which may influence sanitation behaviour. It is not only social identity but also the occupational identity of households that may be linked with norms. Hence, the main occupation of the household may impact sanitation behaviour. Social norms may highly influence households engaged in a traditional occupation, such as farming, due to their extended and deep-rooted networks in the local area. They depend on these networks for their livelihood. On the contrary, households engaged with non-agriculture may have more links with urban centres and therefore not depend on local networks.

The government may play a significant role in behaviour change in sanitation. Along with subsidies, information, education, and communication (IEC) campaigns are one of the necessary means to change people's attitudes and encourage them to use the toilet. In addition, public action is also crucial for developing social infrastructure. Public action may also depend on households' caste and religious identities and people's occupations. The political economy involving social identity and economic prowess may play a significant role in the households' essential service provision (such as water supply) (O'Reilly & Dhanju, 2014; De & Nag, 2016; De, 2009). Access to essential services may, in turn, affect toilet use. The government may also play a significant role in employment and income generation. The latter can impact toilet use positively.

The demographic composition of the household may also have implications for toilet construction and use. If female members can influence household decisions, a household toilet is more likely to be constructed and used. It is because the prime beneficiary of toilet use is female members, especially from privacy, safety, and security concerns. If there are many potential users in a household, then it is likely that all of them may not be able to use it simultaneously. Hence, members of larger households may get dissuaded and may not be able to develop the habit of using the toilet. Figure 6.1 illustrates the drivers impacting toilet use.

Access to Toilet by Religion and Castes

The access to a toilet was very similar across religions. While 67% of Hindus and Christians had access to a toilet, the access was slightly lower at 63% for Muslims. The use of the toilet by all members of households with toilet access demonstrates a different scenario. While all members in 67% of Hindu households use the toilet, it is higher at 71% for Muslim households and 75% for Christian Households. Lesser use of the toilet by Hindu households could be due to religious norms. In Bihar, where a substantial proportion of Muslims was present in the sample, Muslim households had lower access to the toilet than the Hindus (Figure 6.2). However, the percentage of households where all members use the toilet was similar among Hindus and Muslims. In Telangana, access to a toilet is higher for Muslim households than the Hindu and Christian households in the sample. The use of toilets by all members

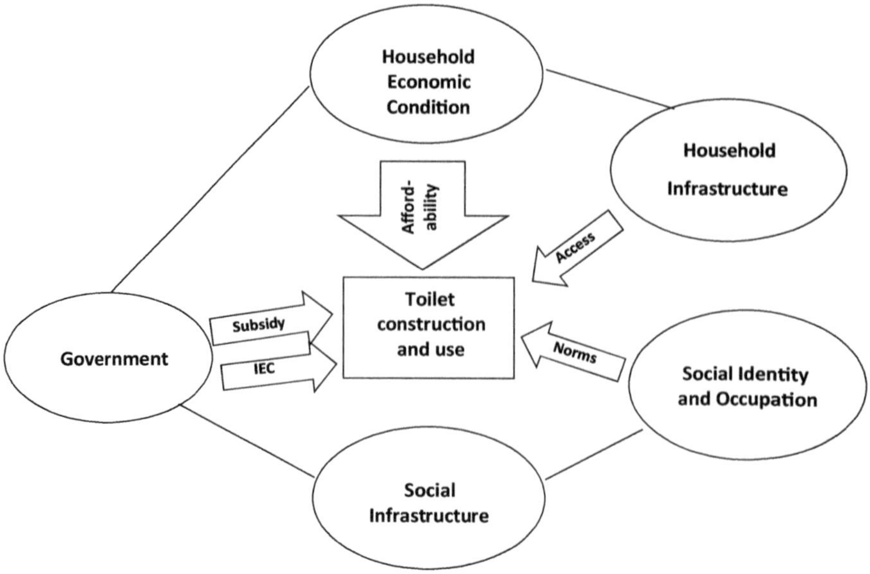

Figure 6.1 Drivers of Toilet Construction and Use.

Source: Authors

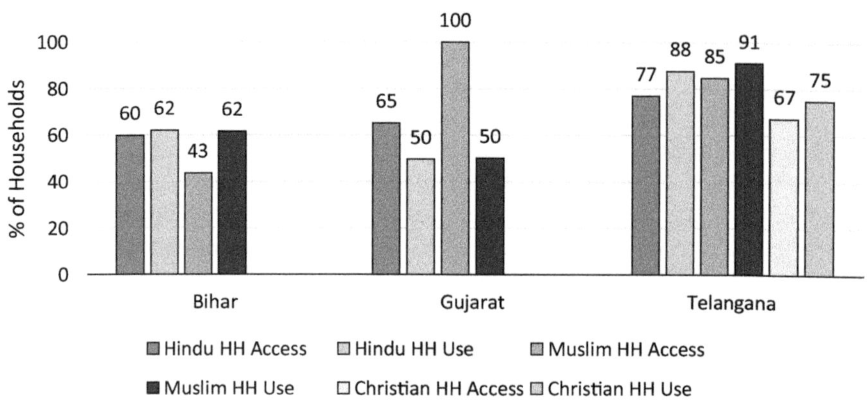

Figure 6.2 All Household Members' Access and Use of Toilets by Religion.

Source: Primary Survey

was also higher in Muslim households than in Hindu households. We cannot make a reasonably good comparison of access and use of the toilet by Hindus and Muslims in Gujarat as the sample of Muslims in Gujarat was lower than in the other two states. In Gujarat, only in half of the households, all members use the toilet.

The analysis of access to a toilet by castes reveals that access is much higher for the upper castes than for other backward castes (Table 6.1). On the contrary, the

Table 6.1 Percentage of Households Having Access to Toilet and Using it (All Members) by Castes

State	*District*	*Upper (General) Castes*		*Backward Castes*					
				Scheduled Caste		*Scheduled Tribe*		*Other Backward Caste*	
		Access	*Use*	*Access*	*Use*	*Access*	*Use*	*Access*	*Use*
Bihar	Sitamarhi	95.24	43.90	74.19	61.84	81.82	66.67	62.65	57.69
	Samastipur	92.86	57.14	37.29	65.15	42.86	71.43	41.10	77.78
	All	94.64	47.27	53.55	63.38	66.67	68.75	52.56	67.01
Gujarat	Sabarkantha			88.61	46.88	82.98	60.61	79.22	50.00
	Dahod			28.95	22.22	51.79	50.00		
	All			69.23	43.84	58.60	54.32	79.22	50.00
Telangana	Medak	95.00	94.74	97.10	92.65	76.92	66.67	98.99	89.80
	Vikarabad	75.00	70.00	57.89	80.85	28.57	100.00	52.83	80.36
	All	87.50	86.21	76.55	67.58	60.00	58.56	75.12	73.31
Overall sample		92.05	60.71	64.48	67.58	59.29	58.56	67.81	73.31

Source: Primary Survey

use of the toilet by all household members was lower in upper caste households. Upper castes may find it challenging to get rid of cultural norms of purity as they may perceive that they are the prime custodian of social norms.

Higher access and lower use of the toilet by upper castes hold in both Bihar and Telangana. The sample did not cover any upper caste household in Gujarat. Within backward castes, access to toilets and their use was lower for scheduled tribes (STs). But the overall pattern does not hold for individual districts. While in Dahod and both the districts of Bihar, STs had better access to toilets than backward castes, in Sabarkantha, the scheduled caste (SC) households had better access than STs.

Regarding the use of the toilet, in all these districts, the use of the toilet by all members was higher for STs than for SCs. The number of ST sample households was significantly less in both the districts of Telangana. Hence, we will not be able to make any robust inference regarding the comparison of the use of toilets between SC and ST households in this state.

The complex dynamics of castes, economic well-being, and living standards vary across the districts. Religious activities were given much more importance than toilet construction in the states. Temples, fairs, or social gatherings were ranked higher in importance than toilets. In the Konaipally village of Telangana, each household contributed Rs. 10000 or more for temple construction, but they could not afford a toilet at home.

Economic Conditions

The per capita expenditure has captured the economic condition of the households. We have segmented the households by per capita expenditure quartiles. Thus, these groups represent different economic classes. The lowest economic class is represented by a per capita monthly expenditure of less than Rs. 725, while the highest economic class is represented by a per capita monthly expenditure of more than Rs. 1925. The percentage of households with access to a toilet was higher in the highest economic class than in the lowest. Still, the increase was not gradual over the economic classes (Table 6.2). Barring Dahod district, none of the districts demonstrated a steady increase in access to a toilet by economic classes. Moreover, in Samastipur and Medak districts, the percentage of households having access to a toilet was not higher in the highest economic class than in the lowest economic class. This analysis implies that economic strength may play an essential role in access to the toilet, but there are other important factors. If the economic conditions had played a significant role, then the access to toilets would have increased with higher economic classes. In this backdrop, Dahod is one district where the economic condition of households plays the most critical role. The migration of households had also dampened the urge to construct a toilet. In Sabarkantha, the priority for the toilet was lowered due to seasonal migration to nearby cities like Ahmedabad and Surat.

All household members' use of the toilet was highest in the lowest economic class and decreased gradually with upgradation to higher and higher economic

Table 6.2 Percentage of Households Having Access to Toilet and Using it (All Members) by Economic Class

State	*District*	*Expenditure Quartiles*							
		Quartile 1		*Quartile 2*		*Quartile 3*		*Quartile 4*	
		(≤Rs. 725)		*(Rs. 725–Rs. 1200)*		*(Rs. 1200–Rs. 1925)*		*(>Rs. 1925)*	
		Access	*Use*	*Access*	*Use*	*Access*	*Use*	*Access*	*Use*
Bihar	Sitamarhi	62.50	30.00	58.70	62.50	79.45	60.66	83.33	58.46
	Samastipur	42.86	84.38	45.16	71.79	39.62	59.38	41.82	58.62
	All	51.35	63.46	50.93	67.61	62.70	60.22	66.17	58.51
Gujarat	Sabarkantha	80.00	62.50	70.21	54.84	80.00	44.44	93.68	51.22
	Dahod	33.87	33.33	47.06	45.83	59.52	53.85	70.59	50.00
	All	40.28	45.00	55.30	50.91	70.65	46.94	90.18	51.11
Telangana	Medak	96.25	91.25	100.00	94.74	94.44	88.24	95.65	84.44
	Vikarabad	52.27	89.36	51.52	63.16	59.32	77.14	61.90	78.57
	All	73.21	90.55	77.78	84.21	72.63	82.61	85.07	83.05
Overall sample		60.51	78.89	58.97	67.76	68.05	64.45	78.85	61.73

Source: Primary Survey

classes. It could be a poorer attempt to use the toilet more than those who are comparatively less poor. The poorer households may have valued infrastructure developed under public programmes more than affluent households. However, the district-wise patterns differ from the overall scenario. The major exception to this pattern is Dahod and Sitamarhi. The exception could be due to the unavailability of other infrastructure such as water supply. Both the districts have a low percentage of households having access to piped water supply in their dwellings. Dahod district had the lowest access to the bathroom for exclusive use.

Social Infrastructure

The use of toilets is crucially dependent on water availability for all household activities such as drinking, cooking, washing, bathing, etc. Piped water supply provides easy and reliable access to the water. Access to piped water supply in dwellings reduced the drudgery of carrying water from elsewhere. Hence, toilet use will likely improve with access to the piped water supply. Overall, access to the toilet and its use improves with the access to piped water supply within the dwelling for household activities. It holds in both Bihar and Gujarat sample districts (Table 6.3). However, it does not hold in Telangana, implying that water availability for a household is a significant constraint for Bihar and Gujarat but not for Telangana. However, the use of a toilet by all household members improves with the access to piped water supply in Telangana, especially in the Medak district. Hence, access to piped water supply in the dwelling improves access to the toilet or its use.

The availability of sufficient water was a significant constraint for the residents of Dahod. Poor households constructed a small water tank in front of their dwelling. Water filled in these tanks was used for household chores. In Telangana, Mission Bhagiratha made water available to the communities and eliminated village water shortages. Every household was provided with a separate water connection outside the dwelling. However, there were exceptions, such as Lingampally in the Vikarabad district, where households faced acute water shortages. At the time of the survey, the used water supply of Rs. 20 per month for two hours per day was stopped. Then they depended on the sole water tank in the village and agricultural bores. These sources were used for drinking and household chores. Water charges vary across villages. Households in Madaram village in Vikarabad used to pay Rs. 40 per month for a one-hour water supply in the morning every day.

Household Infrastructure

Infrastructure in the household has implications for the construction and use of a toilet. The priority of toilet was much lower than other necessitates such as own house with adequate facilities. If the basic construction and facilities available at the house are poor, the household will not likely construct a toilet. There should be a separate space available for bathing and other private activities. Table 4.11 illustrates availability and access to the bathroom. If such space and infrastructure are unavailable, households may not construct toilets. Households may have priorities in their mind, according to which a bathroom for exclusive use may precede the

Table 6.3 Social and Household Infrastructure and Access to Toilets

State	*District*	*Piped Water Supply in Dwelling*				*Bathroom for Household's Exclusive Use*			
		Not Available (%)		*Available(%)*		*Not Available (%)*		*Available (%)*	
		Access to Toilet	*Use of Toilet*	*Access to Toilet*	*Use of Toilet*	*Access to Toilet*	*Use of Toilet*	*Access to Toilet*	*Use of Toilet*
Bihar	Sitamarhi	73.78	58.05	100	0.0	67.4	56.92	100	56.25
	Samastipur	39.9	69.92	100	55.6	26.95	79.31	100	48.89
	All	57.71	62.96	100	38.5	47.99	65.90	100	52.69
Gujarat	Sabarkantha	69.77	60.71	87.5	48.8	65.06	56.52	96.67	48.65
	Dahod	45.45	50.00	100	14.3	47.95	50.00	45.71	33.33
	All	49.79	53.85	88.1	47.1	53.54	53.41	85.16	46.83
Telangana	Medak	100	62.50	96.37	91.0	73.91	76.19	99.44	91.48
	Vikarabad	80	88.89	53.93	79.2	2.17	14.29	100	84.26
	All	88.89	76.47	75.26	86.8	16.52	60.71	99.65	88.73
Overall sample		55.75	61.73	79.65	73.2	44.91	62.16	95.51	71.57

Source: Primary Survey

construction of a toilet. Unavailability of space for toilet construction is also a significant concern in Bihar and Telangana. Our analysis reveals that access to toilets increased with bathroom availability for exclusive use in all three states. Table 6.3 illustrates access to the toilet when the bathroom for exclusive use is available and when it is not. Access to toilets improved with access to the complete bathroom in all the districts barring Dahod. The economic condition of households and access to the piped water supply at the dwelling might have been major constraining factors in the Dahod district. The use of toilets did not increase with access to the bathroom for exclusive use in all districts of Bihar and Gujarat. Only in Telangana, use has increased with access to the complete bathroom. A significant improvement in toilet access and use was observed in Vikarabad, where a bathroom was available for exclusive use for the household members. Economic constraints and availability of piped water in the dwelling were not major constraining factors in this district.

Due to the lack of primary household infrastructure, households put toilets for other types of uses. Households use toilets for activities for which they were not built. In Gujarat's Dahod, households were found using toilets to wash clothes, store fodder, and clean utensils. In Telangana's Vikarabad, toilets were found to be filled with stones. The use of the toilet for bathing and cleaning was also observed in Telangana. The analysis implies that constraints of economic conditions, social infrastructure, and household infrastructure all play essential roles in access to toilets and their use. Still, different constraints may be binding in different places.

Expenditure on Toilets and Government Subsidy

Under the SBM, the government provides a subsidy of Rs. 12000 per household for toilet construction. Our survey reveals that the households may not have received the amount or partially under the programme. Furthermore, although the government provides uniform subsidies across the states, the expenses for the construction of toilets, including labour and material costs, vary across states and districts (Table 6.4). While the average expenses are highest in Bihar, it is lowest in Telangana. The varied expenses for toilet construction across districts were due to differences in sanitary materials and labour costs. It implies that a uniform subsidy across the nation may not be covering costs equally across states. The subsidy amount should be aligned with the local cost structures.

The government subsidy should be able to cover a large proportion of the total expenses of toilet construction. We observe a negative relation between the percentage of toilet construction expenses covered by subsidy in a state and the percentage of households not having access to toilets (Figure 6.3). It implies that states with a lower percentage of toilet construction expenses being covered by subsidy also had a higher percentage of households with no toilet access. Higher access to sanitation in Telangana is associated with subsidy covering more than 95% of toilet construction expenses. Hence, government subsidies must cover a large proportion of toilet construction costs, which may increase toilet construction and access.

Table 6.4 Average Expenditure for Toilet Construction and Average Receipt of Government Subsidy

State	*District*	*Average Expenses (Rs.)*
Bihar	Sitamarhi	44542
	Samastipur	27902
	Total	38118
Gujarat	Sabarkantha	30291
	Dahod	15050
	Total	25719
Telangana	Medak	11880
	Vikarabad	12028
	Total	11934
All		26298

Source: Primary Survey

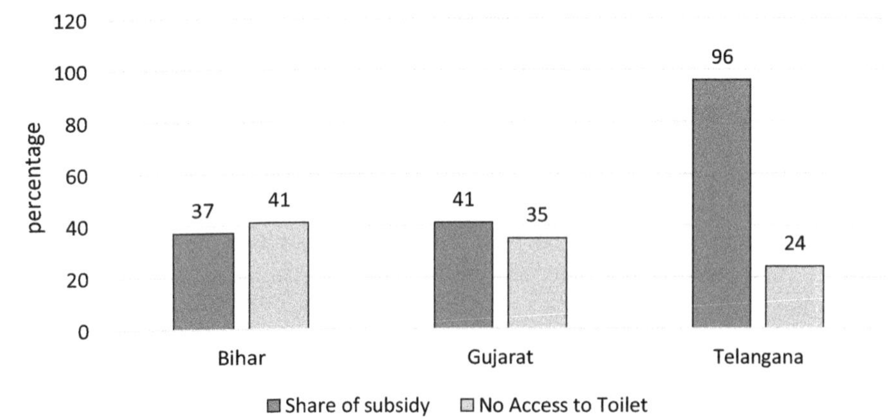

Figure 6.3 Share of Subsidy on Average Expenses and Proportion of Households Having No Access to Toilet.

Source: Primary Survey

Determinants of Access and Use of Toilets

The determinants of having no toilet access, access to toilets for exclusive use, and toilet use by household members are analysed using the multivariate regression analysis. The independent variables are a mix of continuous, discrete, and dichotomous variables, as mentioned below. Religion and state are control variables in the regression model. The dependent variables are no access to a toilet (open defecation), access to the toilet for the household's exclusive use, and actual use of the toilet by the household member(s). These variables are dichotomous, and hence logistic regression model has been used. The details of the regression models are given in the Annexure.

The independent variables capture demography, economic strength, ethnic identity, and others. The larger the household size, the lesser the possibility of toilet construction and use (De, 2018); a single toilet in a large household is not convenient for all the household members. The demand for safe sanitation facilities in rural India is very high from women (Khanna & Das, 2016). Hence, female-headed households are more likely to construct and use the toilet. Due to concerns over privacy, embarrassment, and insecurity, females are more inclined towards the use of the toilet (Simiyu, 2016; De, 2018). Results on attitude towards sanitation also indicated that shame and safety had the highest average agreement score among all the 20 items used to measure attitude towards sanitation. Income, caste, and education significantly impact access to improved toilets in India (Tiwari & Nayak, 2017). The higher the household's total expenditure, the more likely it is for the household to access the toilet and use it. Here, total expenditure is considered an indicator of household income. The land possessed by households is also likely to impact toilet access and use positively.

The higher the percentage of expenses on durable goods and entertainment, the more likely the households are economically better off and would have better access to the toilet. They are more likely to use the toilet as well. Households from backward castes are less likely to construct and use the toilet. Education level is likely to impact access and use of the toilet positively. Better living standards, captured by a house's construction material or a bathroom, are likely to impact toilet construction and use positively.

Along with household infrastructure, availability and access to water are some of the most critical determinants of toilet construction and use (De, 2018; O'Reilly & Louis, 2014). Insufficient water supply for household chores or a higher distance for drinking water is more likely to impact toilet construction and use negatively. Salaried primary earning members are more exposed to the outer world and have better living standards; hence they are more likely to construct and use the toilet. On the other hand, those self-employed in agriculture or non-agriculture are less likely to construct and use toilets.

The likelihood of toilet construction and its use would increase with more information and awareness. Higher person-to-person contact and involvement of people in engendering sanitation programmes may positively impact toilet construction and use (O'Reilly & Louis, 2014; Khanna & Das, 2016). Therefore, awareness about SBM will likely impact toilet construction and use positively. It may be influenced by any other person barring self and spouse. The use of a toilet would also depend on the quality of access to the toilet. If the toilet is for exclusive use, then household members are more likely to use it. Women prefer toilets for exclusive use rather than the toilet that is shared with the neighbours (Simiyu, 2016). Government subsidy may make toilet construction easier but not its use. Toilet use requires behaviour change which may not happen when government subsidy is used for toilet construction. If households are affected by health problems such as flies, stomach upset, or skin disease, they are likely to choose toilet use due to health concerns. The equation and complete explication of the model are presented in Annexure I. Here we present the results of the multiple regression model.

Regression Results

The results of the regression models have been analysed by discussing the impact of variables found statistically significant at 1%, 5%, and 10% levels. The results about access to toilets and the use of toilets have been discussed separately.

Access to Toilet

The regression results about access to toilets are illustrated in Table 6.5.

When **no access to a toilet** (no_access) is the dependent variable, the independent variables with positive significant coefficients are the age of the household head, less than 30 years, Muslim religion, scheduled caste and another backward caste household, a distance of drinking water source 400 meters outside premises, no access to the bathroom, no awareness of SBM, no problem of flies, and state dummies of Gujarat and Telangana. The independent variables having significant negative coefficients are female-headed household, primary occupation self-employed in non-agriculture, religion as Christian, access to a separate bathroom, and no stomach problem in the household. When the availability of a **toilet for exclusive use** (exclusive_toilet) is the dependent variable, then independent variables with positive significant coefficients are other backward castes and upper (general) castes households, access to the primary source of drinking water for household's exclusive use, and total expenses of the household. The independent variables with negative coefficients are drinking water sources outside the dwelling but within the premise, no access to a bathroom, and state dummies of Gujarat and Telangana. All the models can make more than 85% correct predictions.

Table 6.5 Determinants of No Access and Access to Toilets for Exclusive Use

Effect	*Dependent Variables*	
	No Access to Toilet (no_access)	*Exclusive Use of Toilets (exclusive_toilet)*
Positive	HH head age < 30 years*, Muslim religion*, scheduled caste***, other backward caste***, drinking water source outside premises (400 metres and above)**, no bathroom***, no awareness of SBM***, no problem of flies***, Gujarat state***, Telangana state***	Other backward castes*, general (upper) castes***, access to drinking water for HH's exclusive use***, total monthly expenditure of household***
Negative	Female-headed HH*, primary occupation: self-employed in non-agriculture*, Christian religion*, detached bathroom***, total monthly expenditure by household***, no cases of stomach problem*	Drinking water supply source outside dwelling but within premises***, no bathroom***, Gujarat state***, Telangana State***

*significant at 10% level; **significant at 5% level; ***significant at 1% level

The socio-economic background of the households has implications for access to a toilet. The logistic regression analysis results suggest that ethnically backward groups are more likely to practice open defecation. Scheduled castes and other backward castes are more likely to have no access to a toilet. Upper (general) caste households are likelier to have access to a toilet for exclusive use. Muslims (socio-economically backwards) are more likely to have no access to the toilet, while Christians are more likely to have access to toilets than Hindus. Increasing total expenses, an indicator of better economic condition, positively impacts having toilets for exclusive use and harms open defecation. An increase in total expenses by Rs. 1000 per month reduces the chances of open defecation by 1% while increasing toilets for exclusive use by 9%.

Access to the toilet also depends on household leadership and exposure to the outer world. A female-headed household is less likely to continue open defecation, while it is more likely if the head of the household is less than 30 years old. If the primary occupation of the household is self-employed in non-agriculture, then they are less likely to continue open defecation. Access to basic household and social infrastructure impacts access to the toilet. If the household has access to a drinking water facility for exclusive use, it is 14% more likely to have a toilet for exclusive use. If the distance of the drinking water source is more than 400 meters from the premises, then open defecation is more likely by 11% than a drinking water source within the dwelling. If the drinking water source is outside the dwelling but within the premises, then the chances of having toilets for exclusive use go down by 10% compared to within dwelling drinking water source. The bathroom facility plays a vital role in access to the toilet. If the household has no access to the bathroom, then the chances of open defecation increase by 42%, while the chances of the toilet for exclusive use slip by 58%.

If the household is unaware of SBM, the chances of open defecation increase by 10%. If there are no flies in the area, as reported by the household, the chances of open defecation increase by 13%. If the household has better health indicators, such as no stomach problem reported in the last 30 days, it is 5% less likely to go for open defecation. The chances of open defecation are higher by 13% in Gujarat and 30% in Telangana than in Bihar. The chances of having a toilet for exclusive use are lower by 37% in Gujarat and 23% in Telangana than in Bihar.

Regression Results: Use of Toilet

Variables that are found statistically significant in the use of toilets by all the members of the households are presented in Table 6.5. When the toilet used by all male members below 15 years (use_male_below15) is the dependent variable, the coefficient of pucca wall (wall_type_pucca) is significantly positive, and coefficients of the percentage of female at household (per_female), construction of toilet not influenced by self (no_influence_self), and no cases of skin disease (no_skin_disease) at the household are significantly negative (Table 6.6). In the regression taking toilets used by all male members above 15 years (use_male_above15) as the dependent variable, the coefficients of independent variables that are significantly positive

Table 6.6 Determinants of Access to Toilets for Exclusive Use

Effect	*Dependent Variables*				
	use_male_below15	*use_male_above15*	*use_female_below15*	*use_female_above15*	*use_all*
Positive	Wall type: pucca/ concrete***	Primary occupation: self-employed in agriculture***, % of expenses on durable goods and entertainment**	No. of HH members*, highest education of female members in the household – till 10th standard*, wall type: pucca/ concrete*	Highest education of female members in the household – till 10th standard*, primary occupation: service/ salaried*, % of expenses on durable goods and entertainment***, no awareness of SBM**	Bathroom facility detached***, access to toilet exclusively for household***
Negative	% of females in household***, construction of toilet not influenced by self**, no cases of skin disease at household***	No. of household members***, distance of drinking water source – outside premises: 400 metres andabove*,construction of toilet not influenced by self***, construction of the toilet is not influenced by spouse***, Gujarat state**	Construction of toilet not influenced by self**, no cases of skin disease at household***	Drinking water source outside dwelling**, floor type: kaccha/not concrete*, construction of toilet not influenced by self**, construction of the toilet is not influenced by spouse*, no cases of skin disease at household*, Gujarat state**	No. of HH members***, % of female members in household*, construction of toilet not influenced by self***

*significant at 10% level; **significant at 5% level; ***significant at 1% level

are non-agriculture as a primary occupation (primary_occu_self_emp_agri) and percentage expenses on durable goods and entertainment (per_expense_durgood_enter), while the significantly negative coefficients are the total number of household members (total_member), construction of toilet not influenced by self and spouse (no_influence_self no_influence_spouse), and state dummy of Gujarat. When toilet used by all female members below 15 years (use_female_below15) is the dependent variable, the coefficients of the total number of members (total_member), highest education of female members (education_female) as till 10th standard, and pucca wall (wall_type_pucca) are significantly positive, while the coefficients of construction of toilet not influenced by self (no_influence_self) and no cases of skin disease (no_skin_disease) at the household are significantly negative. The coefficients of independent variables such as highest education of female (memberseducation_female) as till 10th standard, salaried household (primary_occu_salary), per percentage of expenses on durable goods and entertainment (expense_durgood_enter), and no awareness of SBM at the household (no_awareness_SBM) are positive and significant in case toilet used by all female above 15 years (use_female_above15) is the dependent variable. The coefficients of independent variables such as drinking water source outside dwelling but within premises, distance of drinking water source (distance_drinking_water) 400 meters and above, construction of toilet not influenced by self (no_influence_self), and state dummy of Gujarat are negative and significant when the same variable as the dependent variable. The percentage of correct prediction is more than 90% in all the models.

In the logistic regression where old-aged members use the toilet (use_old) is the dependent variable, the significant independent variables all have negative coefficients. These variables are the highest education of females till 10th standard, and 10th standard and above, the primary occupation is self-employment in non-agriculture, insufficient availability of water for household chores, a wall made by pucca material, construction of toilet is not influenced by self, the spouse does not influence the construction of the toilet, no problem of flies at the household, and state dummy of Gujarat. When the toilet is used by all members of the household (use_all) is the dependent variable, the significant variables are the total number of members in the household, percentage of females in the household, separate bathrooms, construction of toilets not influenced by self, and access to the toilet for the exclusive use of the household. All the independent variables have negative coefficients, barring detached bathrooms and access to the toilet for the exclusive use of the household. The models are very well fitted. The percentage of correct prediction is more than 90% in all the models, barring the one where the dependent variable is use_old. The latter model makes a 77% correct prediction.

Further, the logistic regression analysis results revealed that a household's demographic and socio-economic characteristics impact the use of the toilet. The larger the household size, the lower the chances of male members above 15 years using it. But, it also leads to a higher chance of toilet use by females below 15 years. Larger households have fewer changes in all the members using the toilet. A 1% increase in female members in the household shows that the chances of male members below 15 years using toilets are lowered by 32%.

Furthermore, a 1% increase in female members in households is likely to reduce all members using the toilet by 23%. Suppose the highest educated female has attended school till 10th standard. There are higher chances of using the toilet for female members below 15 years and above 15 years compared to the household where female members are illiterate. Male members above 15 years of agricultural households are more likely to use the toilet. The household economic condition has a high impact on toilet use. A 1% increase in expenses on durable goods increases the chances of using toilets for males and females above 15 years by 44% and 52%, respectively.

Both household and social infrastructure have implications for toilet use. The longer the distance travelled to fetch drinking water, the lesser the chances of toilet usage among females above 15 years: the chances reduce by 9% if the source is outside the dwelling but within premises and 15% if the source is away by more than 400 metres (Table 6.7). Usage of the toilet for males above 15 years also reduces by 12% if the source of drinking water is away by 400 meters and above. A bathroom separate from the house that is not attached to the living or bedroom increases the chances of toilet use by all household members. Access to the toilet for the exclusive use of the household increases the chance of all household members using it by 14%. Housing condition, which is an indicator of the standard of living, has implications for toilet usage. Brick-and-mortar walls (*pucca*) increases the chances of using the toilet by male below 15 years and female below 15 years. Similarly, a mud floor (*kutcha*) reduces the chances of toilet use by females above 15 years.

The influences of respondents (69% are head of household) and their spouses have a very high impact on the usage of toilets. The influence of the household head on toilet construction increases the chances of toilet use for all age groups and gender. The influence of spouses on toilet construction increases the chances of toilet use for male and female members older than 15 years of age. Concerning health and hygiene conditions, if skin disease is prevalent, there is a higher likelihood of using the toilet by males and females below 15 years and females above 15 years. The likelihood of toilet use is generally lower in Gujarat for male and female household members above 15 years than for respective household members in Bihar.

Rounding It Up

We have attempted to find the major determinants of access and use of toilets. Household's socio-economic conditions, social identity, occupation, household infrastructure, social infrastructure, and government intervention are considered as determinants. We found that access to toilets was similar across different religions but the use of toilets by all members was higher for Muslims and Christians as compared to Hindus. We also found that access was higher for upper castes but the use of toilets by all members of household was lower for upper caste households. The norms of purity for Hindu upper castes may have affected toilet use adversely.

Access to toilets is better for higher economic class households. But access does not increase with the rising economic class always. This implies that along with the economic condition of households other factors play crucial roles in toilet access. More surprisingly, the use of toilets by all members of households was best in the

Table 6.7 Determinants of Usage of Toilet

Effect	*Dependent Variables*				
	use_male_below15	*use_male_above15*	*use_female_below15*	*use_female_above15*	*use_all*
Positive	Wall type: pucca/ concrete***	Primary occupation: self-employed in agriculture***, % of expenses on durable goods and entertainment**	No. of HH members*, highest education of female members in household – till 10th standard*, wall type: pucca/ concrete*	Highest education of female members in household – till 10th standard*, primary occupation: service/ salaried*, % of expenses on durable goods and entertainment***, no awareness of SBM**	Bathroom facility detached***, access to toilet exclusively for household***
Negative	% of female in household***, construction of toilet not influenced by self**, no cases of skin disease at household***	No of household members***, distance of drinking water source – outside premises: 400 metres andabove*,construction of toilet not influenced by self***, construction of the toilet is not influenced by spouse***, Gujarat state**	Construction of toilet not influenced by self**, no cases of skin disease at household***	Drinking water source outside dwelling**, floor type: kuccha/not concrete*, construction of toilet not influenced by self**, construction of the toilet is not influenced by spouse*, no cases of skin disease at household*, Gujarat state**	No. of HH members***, % of female members in household*, construction of toilet not influenced by self***

*significant at 10% level; **significant at 5% level; ***significant at 1% level

lowest economic class and decreased gradually with higher and higher economic class. This implies that the poorer households value toilets more than the richer households once toilets are built. The higher the government subsidy amount in meeting total toilet construction expenses, the lesser the lack of access. Along with economic conditions, access to piped water supply in dwellings improves access to toilets and their use. Similarly, access to bathrooms for households' exclusive use also improves toilet access and use. However, these constraints of economic conditions and infrastructure need not be binding everywhere at the same time; different constraints are binding in different places at a time.

The regression results illustrate the major determinants of toilet access and use. The economic strength of households has a significant positive impact on access and use. Hence, government subsidies or incentives may help in toilet construction. The living standard of households has a significant impact on both access and use of the toilet. The results reveal that having no bathroom, having no access to an exclusive source of drinking water, and greater distances from the drinking water source are detrimental to having toilets for the exclusive use of toilets. More specifically, greater distances from the water supply source significantly reduce the toilet use by a female. The drudgery of fetching water from outside may have discouraged the female from using the toilet.

The type of structure of the house has profound implications on the usage of the toilet. Hence, sanitation coverage and behavioural change are possible to usher in through holistic improvement of living standards, not just toilet construction through public programmes. Social norms of cleanliness and family norms intertwined with house structure may impact toilet use. Households having detached bathrooms are more likely to use toilets by all members than households having bathrooms attached to bedrooms or living rooms.

Awareness of SBM reduces the chances of open defecation by 10%. Yet, the influence of health or social workers is not significant. The household heads and their spouses have a significant influence on the use of the toilet, especially for the adult. Hence, social communication regarding behavioural change may be targeted to adult male and female decision-makers of households. As the prevalence of skin disease is one of the triggers of toilet use by the younger population, with whom behaviour change can have a long-lasting effect and can also have an impact on older generations, public programmes for sanitation should target communities where such disease is prevalent.

The regression results also suggest that the design of one toilet per household in a public sanitation programme is detrimental to toilet use in larger households. Female members are given priority over and above male members if the total number of household members is high or the percentage of female members in the household is high. Hence, sanitation programmes should plan to construct multiple toilets in larger households.

Note

1 https://www.worldbank.org/en/topic/sanitation#1.

7 Public Action

Small collectives and external funding play a crucial role in sustaining behaviour change. This chapter also discusses that one major impediment to behaviour change is the target-driven construction of toilets. Although sanitation is a private behaviour, it has public implications too. Qualitative tools and techniques were used to explore and understand the individual and the group's behaviour towards sanitation. Focused group discussions (FGDs), participatory rural appraisals (PRAs), unstructured interviews, and Zaltman Metaphor Elicitation Technique (ZMET) were used and conducted with and by the community. It helped us understand the sociocultural structure, natural and physical resources, presence and role of collectives, and public and private institutions. Furthermore, caste composition, gender roles, social norms, social awareness, public initiatives, perception, and household preferences were essential for sanitation behaviour. Each tool and technique was unique and steered to explore and triangulate the qualitative data and information of the existing social structure of the selected region.

Focused group discussions with small-sized exclusive groups, usually seven to eight members of men, women, youths, Self-Help Group (SHG), and social action committee, have helped build rapport with the community. They have also helped form trust and clarify the objectives and purpose of the research and field survey. During the discussions, it was communicated that the respondent's personal and private identity would not be disclosed to any private or public entities. Participatory rural appraisal involves the community members, such as men, women, differently abled, youth, children, and community representatives and leaders. FGDs, followed by PRA, enabled community mobilisation and engagement. The exercise was unique and exciting, thus refraining community members from dispersing and accelerating to contribute their knowledge and experience of the locality. Unstructured or informal interviews with masons, Panchayat members, ZMET, and household surveys enabled us to analyse the conscious and subconscious sociocultural and psychological realities of the households in the rural set-up. Thus, these tools were essential to tap the perceptions, preferences, barriers, and needs of different sections of society to have a holistic view of sanitation.

DOI: 10.4324/9781032726267-7

Participatory Rural Appraisal

A participatory rural appraisal (PRA) is an approach and method for learning about rural life and conditions through rural people. PRA is a set of approaches and methods to enable rural people to share, enhance, and analyse their knowledge of life and conditions, plan, and act. The PRA approach became popular in the 1990s, shifting from a 'top-down' to a 'bottom-up' approach in planning. In PRA, villagers organise local knowledge and information and present it cohesively with an indigenous flavour. The methodology can help collect data, identify and mobilise intended groups, and evoke their participation. Intended groups can participate in decision-making, project design, implementation, and monitoring. It provides an alternative framework for data collection and analysis. This approach helps focus on people's knowledge and understanding regarding their locality, livelihoods, and interrelationships with socio-economic and ecological factors. The process enables investigation, analysis, and evaluation of constraints and opportunities. It assesses the needs and priorities in agriculture, small-scale rural enterprises, and other social and economic development programmes addressed to village development.

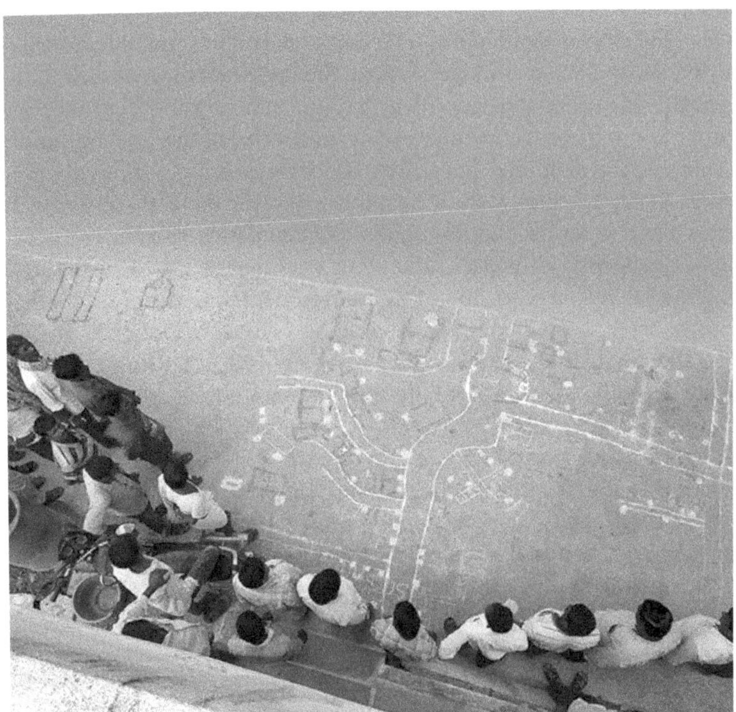

Figure 7.1 Social Mapping.

Source: Author Deepa Gupta

Social and resource mapping (see Figure 7.1) is one of the crucial tools of PRA. Such maps portray the image of houses in a village, their distribution of farms and fields, public and private institutions such as schools, Anganwadi centres, hospitals, Panchayati raj Institutions (PRIs), religious places, post offices, Public Distribution System (PDS), Primary Health Centres (PHCs), local and informal markets, and any other shared places. Mapping can also help depict natural resources, local land use, soil classifications, rivers, drainage points, and boundaries with other villages. The map is usually prepared with the community's help, including children (see Figure 7.1). Transect walk through the fields and the village, viewing the area from a high vantage point, could help produce social and resource maps. It is also known as a base map and helps understand the villages' diversity. This process also helps build rapport with the community and makes them comfortable sharing and discussing their knowledge and experience of their villages. Mapping can be done in any suitable and commonplace where everyone from the community could reach and gather to share and execute the process (see Figure 7.1). The place is usually selected in consultation with the community members after discussing the purpose of tools and approaches. Mapping on the ground could be visible to people as they may draw with the help of chalk, coloured powder, pebbles of different sizes, wood pieces, leaves, etc. Mapping the resources with and by the community is an art and an enthusiastic experience. The place where it is usually performed is a vast canvas. The role of facilitator or researcher becomes crucial to coordinate and facilitate diverse artists, i.e., villagers' ideas and understanding of their village. The advantages of such approaches are that they generate a good deal of information in less time; allow discussions, alterations, and corrections, are fun and precise; and are valuable for planning, implementation, monitoring, and evaluation. Once the villagers make a social map, it becomes easy for them to describe locations within the village in terms of household's characteristics in terms of accessibility to resources, ownership of houses, and other vital features. In a resource map, the villagers draw the resource profile of the village depicting different kinds of soils, rivers, ponds, trees, crops, community grazing land, threshing yard, agricultural produce, market, irrigation source, agricultural inputs depot, topography, etc. Thus, the resource map allows to explore the development challenges and opportunities in the villages.

Furthermore, participatory transect walks systematically involve walking with the villagers through an area and discussing different aspects of land-use agro-ecological zones in the village observed during the walk. This PRA method used to explore the spatial dimensions of people's realities. A walk by a PRA team from one point of the village to another enables to observe different types of rural ecology and discuss soil conditions, land use patterns, crops, livestock, fisheries, micro-environments with rural people, agro-ecological zones, etc. Transect reveals villagers' perception of their natural, physical, differing resources, etc. The transect is different from resource mapping. The resource map provides a bird's eye view of the locality. The transect depicts the cross-sectional view of the different agro-ecological zones and provides a comparative assessment of zones of different parameters.

Further, the PRA tools include various other approaches of mapping, diagramming, and ranking such as seasonal calendars, time trends, timelines, mobility maps, analytical games (including techniques such as ranking: preference ranking, pairwise ranking, matrix ranking), wealth ranking, livelihood analysis, Venn diagram, etc. Literature suggests that PRA tools have been broadly used to understand and explore livelihood resources and opportunities in a particular village. They have been used to map various farm, off-farm, and non-farm activities in the village, distribution of agricultural resources, migrants in the household, land ownership, wealth assets, livestock, fisheries, the proportion of income, expenditure, credit, and debt, season-wise variation in earning, consumption pattern, etc (see Figure 7.2). PRA provides scope for all involved to learn from each other and stimulates self-propelled initiatives. The basic principle of PRA states that the process should not be unduly hurried or rushed. It is also essential to triangulate the information through various sources and approaches. The green dots outside the houses represented in Figure 7.2 show that the community preferred to construct the toilet outside the dwelling. Thus, using PRA tools enabled us to explore the villages' existing sanitation facilities and the challenges associated with their accessibility to the rural poor.

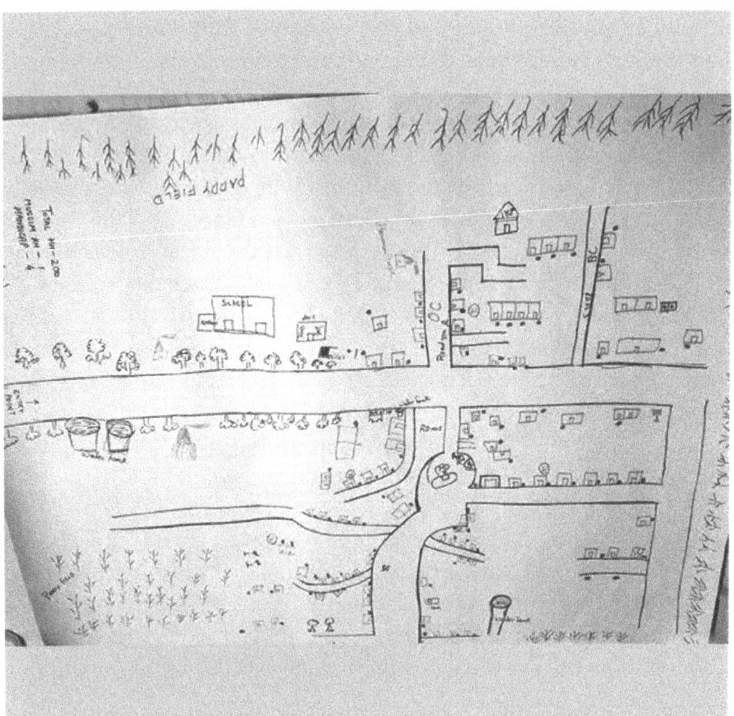

Figure 7.2 Social Map for Sanitation.

Source: Author Deepa Gupta

Role of Gram Panchayat and District Administration

Gram Panchayat and district administration have a crucial role to play in implementing sanitation programmes at the grassroots. The exploratory study suggests that the role of local bodies and administration differs even in the identical institutional set-up. It has been observed that the best-performing districts of Bihar, Gujarat, and Telangana have more significant involvement of district administration at all stages of planning, implementation, and monitoring of sanitation programmes. However, at the same time, it has also been investigated that the better engagement of district and local administration may not have a sustainable approach to implementing public schemes. For instance, Sitamarhi and Samastipur districts were selected as Bihar's best- and least-performing districts. PRI members' and district administration's implementation and monitoring strategies were quite distinctive in these districts regarding promotional activities, incentive disbursement, and community involvement. The district authority of Sitamarhi was passionately invested in achieving all the set targets of SBM(G) in the district; on the other hand, Samastipur was inconsistent, less involved, and less attentive to achieving sanitation targets.

Similarly, Sabarkantha and Dahod were selected as Gujarat's best- and least-performing districts. Due to the geographical and demographical differences, the local and district officials strategised the initiatives differently. Access to information and markets is better for the Sabarkantha community than Dahod. Dahod is a tribal district, and its inhabitants are scattered demographically. It has also been observed that the government officials have less priority in visiting demographically challenged regions and thus shifted the whole focus of implementing SBM(G) to the best-connected districts. During the informal interviews with district officials, it has been explored that lack of skilled labour and far-flung locations are a few of the main factors for low toilet construction and unachieved targets of SBM(G) in Dahod. In Medak, much like the approach in Sitamarhi district, local authorities and leaders have mandated that rural households lacking toilets will not be eligible for various social security and welfare programmes, including PDS, pension, electricity, etc. This measure is implemented to ensure the successful accomplishment of the toilet construction target.

Therefore, Samastipur, Dahod, and Vikarabad exhibit lower levels of Gram Panchayat and district administration engagement compared to the Sitamarhi, Sabarkantha, and Medak districts.

A woman participating in a Focus Group Discussion (FGD) in Dahod asserted, "Local bodies used to visit the village only during elections, and afterward, they tend to forget all their promises." Additionally, it has been observed that districts with improved access to markets, active community involvement, and dedicated government officials exhibit higher awareness and information regarding the construction and usage of toilets.

Medak and Vikarabad have been selected as the best- and least-performing districts in Telangana. District officials of Medak coordinated well with the Gram Panchayat to achieve all the SBM(G) targets and develop the model villages.

Malkapur village of Medak district was declared ODF back in 2016. Masons from neighbouring districts were hired for toilet construction. Toilet was constructed by the masons from the same community in all other blocks. The Panchayat facilitated the construction of toilets, with community organisations actively participating in mobilisation and awareness-building efforts. During the FGD, it was explored that the Panchayat has outsourced the toilet maintenance by appointing a cleaner to clean the household's toilets weekly in the village. They have also directed the rural community to keep their cattle in the agricultural field to maintain cleanliness in the hamlets and prevent unpleasant odours from waste. They believed that keeping livestock within the community could result in excessive waste and obstacles in attaining the cleanliness and hygiene goals of the model village. Consequently, community members have relocated their cattle to the fields, increasing household workload. Local political leaders' engagement level was more pronounced in Telangana villages than in Bihar and Gujarat.

The government official in Wadiyaram mentioned that poor allocation of funds is one of the main reasons for the poor implementation of the programme at the grassroots and hence did not meet the toilet construction targets. It has been noticed that Wadiyaram experienced a relatively significant political influence, with individuals in close proximity to power often exerting dominance in the decision-making process for implementations. FGD and transect walk highlighted some of the community's water and toilet availability concerns. Community members have complained that they still do not have access to piped water at the dwelling. Local body members conveniently tried to escape the situation and justify that it would be done soon.

However, the community became agitated and furious, demanding an immediate solution after enduring a prolonged wait. In contrast, Lingampally achieved ODF status in 2017 and exhibited a more favourable sanitation condition compared to other villages in the Vikarabad district. To promote toilet usage, the community and the PRI members undertook various initiatives, including door-to-door visits, wall paintings (see Figures 7.3 and 7.5), Nukkad Natak, and cultural folk dances. Additionally, Panchayat members have implemented a penalty in the form of a monetary fine for individuals caught practicing open defecation.

Role of Small Collectives

At the grassroots level, small collectives like self-help groups (SHGs), village organisations, cluster-level federations, youth groups, and social action committees play a crucial role in each SBM(G) implementation stage. In Gujarat villages, women's involvement was limited, even when they were the Mahila Mandals (SHGs) members. Conversely, women groups exhibit greater activity in Bihar villages (see Figure 7.4) than in Gujarat. On the contrary, youth groups are more engaged in and committed to activities in Telangana villages than in Bihar and Gujarat. These small collectives typically focus on community mobilisation, raising awareness, providing training, and organising meetings and workshops at the local level.

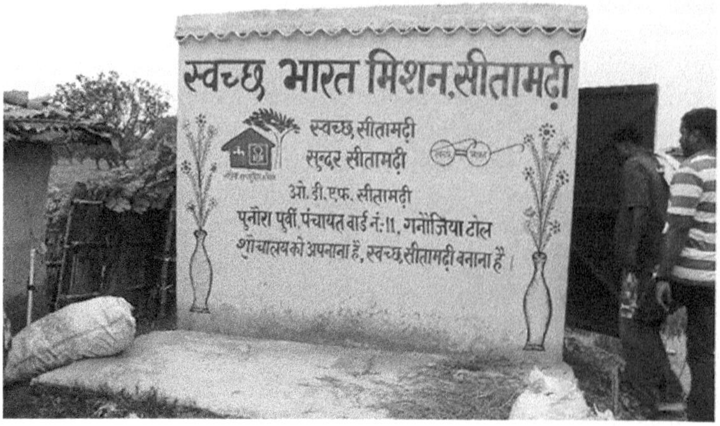

Figure 7.3 Initiative by District Administration.

Source: Author Deepa Gupta

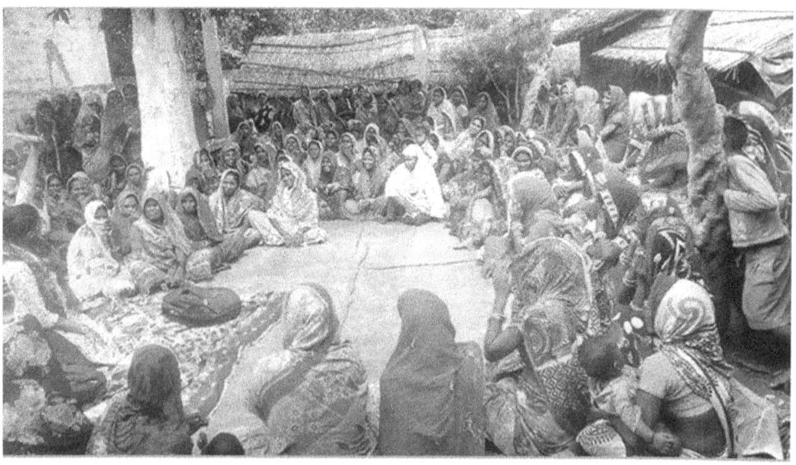

Figure 7.4 Meeting at Village Organisation.

Source: Author Deepa Gupta

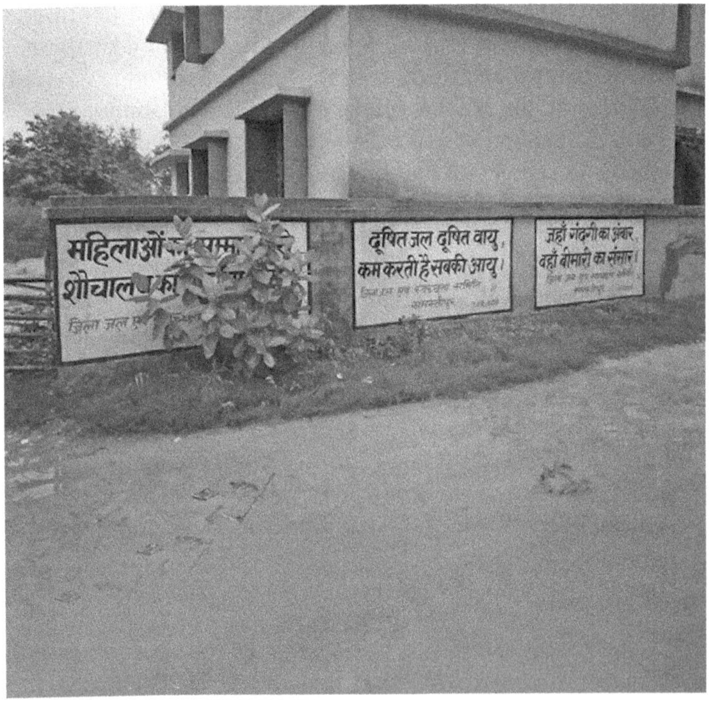

Figure 7.5 Wall Painting.

Source: Author Deepa Gupta

In Bihar, Self-Help Groups (SHGs), Village Organizations, and Cluster Level Federations ensured toilets' construction, while the responsibility for promoting toilet usage fell on the social action committee. In Telangana, active youth groups are involved in community mobilisation and participating in community mobilisation; social action committees in coordination with SHGs are ensuring toilet construction, usage of toilets, and household waste segregation. Youth groups in Telangana villages also maintain comprehensive records related to sanitation. District officials of Gujarat have emphasised that SHGs and Panchayat members must recommend the demand for the toilet in the household. However, field analysis revealed a paradox indicating that the involvement of women groups or SHGs in Gujarat is limited. Thus, unlike Bihar and Telangana, small collectives such as SHGs, social action committees, and youth groups are less active in Gujarat. Panchayat members in Gujarat are primarily responsible for generating toilet demand and overseeing other implementation processes.

Issues of Convergence

The guideline of SBM(G) suggests that convergence of the programme with small collectives such as SHGs, Cluster Level Federations, and government schemes such as MGNREGA and NRLM has vast potential to create livelihoods for the rural poor. Enhancing capacity and empowering the existing institutional network is essential. The Panchayat and district administration have endeavoured to incorporate communities into the mission implementation and planning processes, aiming to optimise the utilisation of available resources. At the same time, it has been observed that the convergence of programmes with other schemes and institutions has diverse challenges. The challenges related to convergence in Telangana differ significantly from those in Bihar. Issues such as delayed fund disbursement, political influence, caste-based politics, and transfer of incentives in multiple installments pose distinct challenges to convergence in Telangana.

Conversely, Gujarat faces a significant challenge with the limited participation of the community and a shortage of skilled labour for toilet construction. In Bihar, community involvement is comparatively higher than in Gujarat, but challenges persist in terms of disseminating information and creating awareness. It has been explored during the community interaction that convergence with NRLM facilitated efficient management at the grassroots. However, at the same time, delays in the disbursement of funds have led to trust issues among community members.

Disbursement of Funds

The qualitative analysis recommends states adopt varied approaches in fund allocation for toilet construction. The rural households of Telangana received an incentive of Rs. 12000 for toilet construction in two equal installments. The initial installments is disbursed upon the completion of twin pits, with the full payment provided only after the entire toilet construction is finished. The Panchayat verifies and reports the progress of toilet construction before fund transfer. In Gujarat and Bihar, the incentive amount has been disbursed only in single installment after verification by the Panchayat and completion of toilet construction. In Bihar, SHG members have taken a loan to construct the toilet from SHGs and Village Organizations from the Sanitation, Hygiene and Nutrition (SHAN) fund. SHAN is a specific sanitation, health, and nutrition fund at Village Organizations under the State Rural Livelihoods Mission. These individuals have constructed their toilets by using their own funds. The social action committee verified and reported the toilet construction in the Panchayat. Furthermore, the incentive amount is disbursed to individual households. SHG members from Sitamarhi and Vikarabad districts have expressed that the incentive amount is insufficient to construct the toilet, attributing it to the rising costs of labour and construction materials. Community members in Bihar have mentioned that the household had received money after constructing the toilet, and at the initial phase, they need money. Consequently, they borrowed money from SHG at a one percent interest rate. Villages of the Sitamarhi district have mentioned that distance from the primary market made transporting construction materials expensive. Similarly, community members from Dahod and Medak have reported that the households have submitted the reimbursement form to the Panchayat but have not received the incentive amount. Thus, the challenges in fund disbursement vary across states and often involve decentralised coping mechanism.

External Funding

The village of Malkapur in the Medak district has been awarded a grant of Rs. 10 lakhs from an international donor for community development. This grant recognises the community's efforts to achieve open-defecation-free status. The Panchayat has decided in collaboration with the community to utilise the funds for enhancing the village's waste disposal system. This includes improving the drainage system, providing separate bins of solid and liquid waste, cleanliness drives, village plantation initiatives, and developing a scenic rock garden for the community. These endeavours collectively contributed to enhancing sanitation, elevating the standard of living for rural households, and promoting overall community well-being. In contrast, SHGs in Bihar have separate funds for sanitation, health, and nutrition (SHAN), and they also set aside separate monthly savings for health-related needs. SHAN funds have been used to construct toilets in rural households. Consequently, both Bihar and Telangana benefit from external funding support to enhance the sanitation status of their villages. This external funding has spurred greater community organisations' involvement in implementing the sanitation programme in both the states of Bihar and Telangana.

Sanitation Campaign

In Bihar, community mobilisation and awareness creation for sanitation has been facilitated through the SHGs and Village Organizations (see Figure 7.4). Simultaneously, the district and local administration were directly involved in implementing SBM(G). Various initiatives such as, morning vigilance, whistle-blowing, meetings, training, workshops, *Tatti par Matti* (cover the shit with soil), Nukkad Natak, door-to-door visits, rallies, wall paintings, billboards, the appointment of *Swacchatagrahi*, etc. have been undertaken to raise awareness and disseminate information to stop open defecation. However, during the FGD, it was observed that some community members were unaware of the sanitation programme. In Telangana, there is a relatively higher awareness of proper sanitation practices among male household members than in Bihar. While women groups in Bihar actively address the villages' social development issues, sanitation still receives lower priority.

Community members are still show limited concern regarding the safe disposal of baby faeces, menstrual hygiene, and the use of the toilet by all household members. The swacchhagrahis is pivotal in facilitating toilet demand to the Panchayat and ensuring seamless disbursements of incentives to the household. It has been observed that the households are aware of the term *Swacchata*, there is a lack of awareness about the swacchhagrahis in the village. Both transect walk and FGDs revealed that lower utilisation of Information, Education and Communication (IEC) material in Gujarat compared to Bihar. Additionally, Dahod, Samastipur, and Vikarabad districts having lower awareness regarding SBM compared to Sabarkantha, Sitamarhi, and Medak districts.

The significant factor contributing to the low awareness among community members is the limited involvement of local and district administration. The community in Sabarkantha responded that television serves as a valuable source of information and their awareness of the Swachh Bharat Mission stems from television broadcast. In Medak, visual and print media actively captured and reported community sanitation efforts. **In Telangana,** the **'Swacchata Hi Sewa'** campaign encouraged community to participate in the cleanliness drive (Swacchata campaign). However, they have also indicated that only a few households had participated, with the majority being unaware of the campaign. Children across villages are the most aware community members and act as crucial messengers to the households (see Figure 7.6). They demonstrated knowledge of village's handwashing practices, toilet usage, and *Swacchata Abhiyan*. Both male and female community members hold diverse views regarding the rewards for using toilets and penalties for non-compliance. Generally, male members were hesitant about imposing penalties for open defecation, although they acknowledged a gradual acceptance of the new behaviour among the people.

On the other hand, the women's groups in the Samastipur district expressed that the felicitation for adopting exemplary sanitation practices could motivate other households in the locality to adopt best practices. Similarly, a female member from Sabarkantha also mentioned that the household must be awarded for the

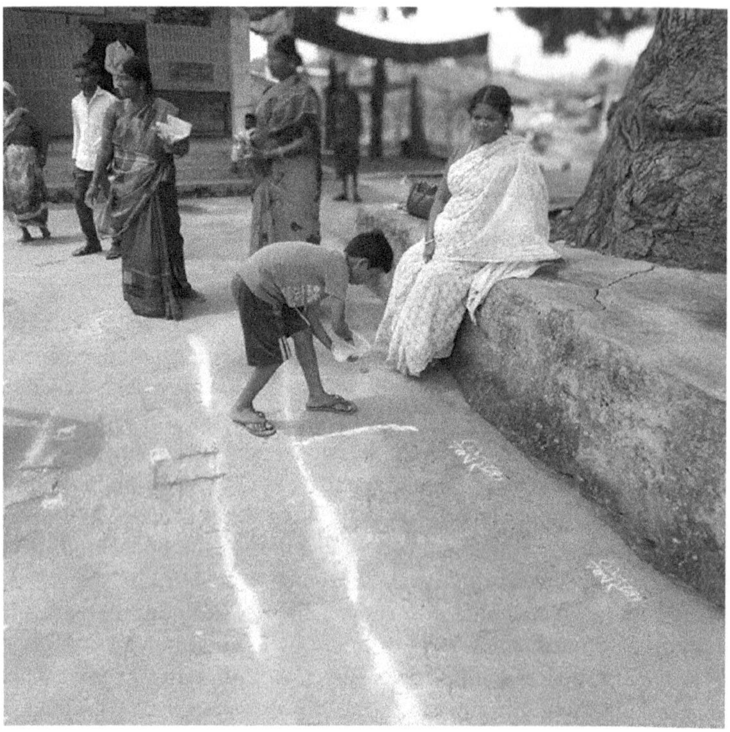

Figure 7.6 Child Participation in PRA.

Source: Author Deepa Gupta

best practices for sanitation. In both Telangana and Bihar, social action committees exhibited increased activity and functionality in villages particularly in conducting morning vigilance to stop open defecation. The initiative was quite effective initially and facilitated the implementation process. Moreover, sustaining regular engagement with the community during unconventional hours became challenging over time. Furthermore, individuals started altering their locations and timings for open defecation, driven by concerns about potential social sanctions or penalties, even after constructing the toilet.

Community Participation

Focused group discussions (FGDs) conducted separately with women and men members of the community to comprehend the gender-specific concerns, priorities, and beliefs regarding sanitation facilities. It has been observed that the participation of the community differs in the villages. It has been explored that the participation of the community in sanitation activities and campaigns depends on various dynamics such as access to public institutions, knowledge and information, social networks, age, caste, gender, and social norms. Participatory Rural Appraisal (PRA) revealed that individuals from lower caste exhibit limited involvement in decision-making processes within the village.

There are incidences where the community subtly expresses a sense of exclusion from the main village, indicating a distinct perception compared to higher castes. During the PRA in Ibrahimpur, Medak district, the higher caste individuals utilised maximum resources including land, chalk, and colour to delineate their hamlets and public institutions In contrast, the scheduled castes' hamlets were depicted with less space and fewer colours. The study delved into the psychological realities of constructing and using the toilet through community participation

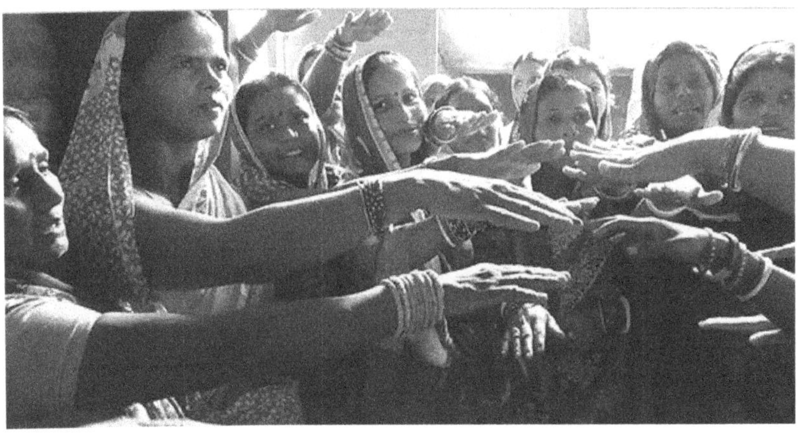

Figure 7.7 Women Taking Oath to Use Toilets.

Source: Author, Deepa Gupta

in representing their physical and social realities. Across the villages, it has been observed that the community predominantly utiliszed mapping materials such as colours, chalk, and physical space, to portray the hamlets and houses of higher caste and hindu religious sites. Conversely, few materials were allocated to represent lower caste hamlets, along with anganwadi, PDS, PHCs, and APHCs.

Thus, during representation, the community predominantly focused on higher caste hamlets, natural resources, agricultural fields, and physical resources, particularly water tanks, Panchayati Raj Institutions (PRIs), and schools. During the process, it has been observed that the size of the represented physical structure, such as church, mosque, and houses of minorities, SCs, and STs, was comparatively smaller. It was also observed that the SC/ST women exclusively drew SC/ST hamlets (see Figure 7.8), while others showed minimal interest in representing their hamlets. Additionally, the youth were more interested in representing schools, colleges, water bodies, agricultural fields, and temples. Simultaneously, the children actively corrected the map, ensuring the accurate inclusion of physical amenities, particularly church, mosque, SC/ST hamlets, and water tanks. Throughout the villages, it has been noticed that the participation of adolescent girls and young or newly wed women was notably lower than that of young boys and older women. Usually, the SC and ST hamlets are at the end of the village and have limited access to resources compared to higher caste households. Compared to other villages of the Vikarabad district, in Neelapally, women actively mobilised community members to share their knowledge and sanitation challenges. Neelapally stood out as the

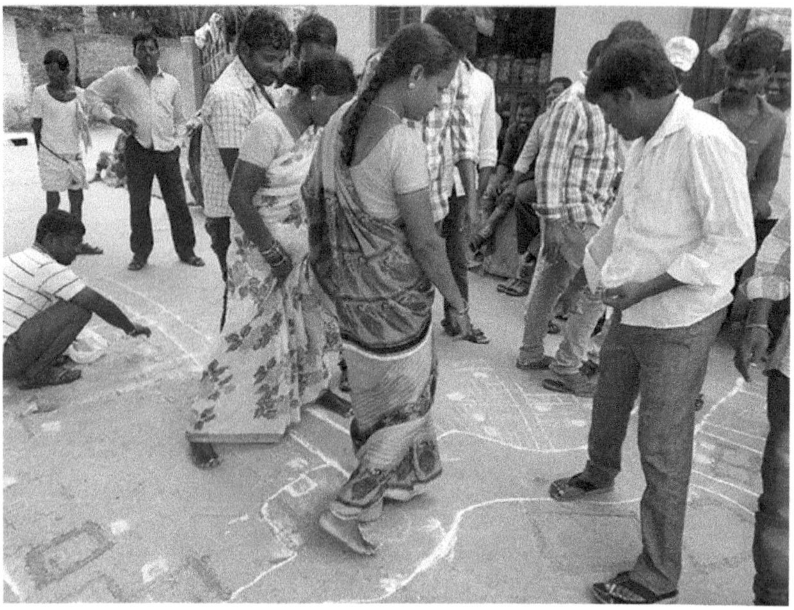

Figure 7.8 Women Representing Sanitation Status.

Source: Author, Deepa Gupta

only village in Telangana where youth participation was low, attributed to lack of awareness and inadequate infrastructure.

Furthermore, in the Rampur village of Samastipur district, the aspiration for improved health and hygiene cannot be achieved with the involvement of only a few households. Therefore, the entire community must come together. Women members of SHGs have emphasised that if '*I have started using the toilet but other members of the society still defecating in the open, then it does not make any sense as we are ultimately contributing to the environmental pollution.*' Separate FGDs with men and women in Bihar have revealed that the prohibition on alcohol has also encouraged community participation in toilet construction. Additionally, individuals have also emphasised establishing a safe waste disposal system. Members from the community stated that 'our village is not so clean, although a few of us have constructed toilets and are using it. Nevertheless, this is not enough, and we require a proper system that must include the responsibility of public administration, community ownership, and resource maintenance responsibilities.' Varied initiatives such as separate dust bins at a commonplace, segregation of waste at the household level, door-to-door waste collection, waste treatment, timely pit emptying, and village cleaning drives are considered essential to maintaining a clean environment. These efforts contribute to public benefits through community engagement.

The migration of rural men to urban areas for improved livelihood opportunities has exposed them to urban and semi-urban amenities and lifestyles. The migration has, in turn, left families in rural areas with inadequate health and sanitation infrastructure. The exposure to better sanitation facilities in urban settings has prompted these male migrants to plan and construct basic sanitation structures for their households. They also facilitated community mobilisation and planning for overall community well-being. Malkapur village was developed as a model village with robust community participation. Youth members in the community were very active in the village. They actively participated in and taken sanitation initiatives, such as the village cleaning drive, regular meetings, training, and workshops at the village level. The village-level committee, such as the social action committee, has been formed to take initiatives to monitor and create awareness to stop open defecation. In Malkapur, it was decided to impose a penalty of Rs. 500 per person found guilty of defecating in the open. In Telangana, agricultural field made it easier for households to dispose of waste and practice open defecation.

Furthermore, it has been discussed that community members have changed their timings and places for open defecation due to the apprehension of facing penalties. During the discussion, the social action committee shared that eliminating open defecation from the community is a challenging mission that demands consistent efforts. To address this, the village-level committee initiated *a non-stop sanitation drive* for 30 days, where community members committed to dedicate two hours daily to clean the village. The positive outcome of the initiative taken in Malkapur village started spreading the word of change in the nearby villages, turning Malkapur into a model for development and an improved quality of life. During field visits to Konaipally village in Medak district, a community member expressed, '*we also want the same development as Malkapur, and we will take all such good initiatives to achieve the goal.*' Like Malkapur, community members of Konaipally village have also planned to develop a community park, rename their hamlets, ban alcohol, construct toilets, access piped water supply under Mission Bhagiratha, and organise regular cleanliness drives in the village. The community has taken collective action to ban alcohol in the Toparan block, leading to reduction in domestic violence and community conflicts in the villages. In Imbrahimpur, during the Ganesh Chaturthi, the community contributed to celebrating more than twenty-five Ganesh pandals. In Konaipally, the community contributed Rs. 3 lakhs to build the *Pedamma* temple in the village. Each household of the village contributed Rs. 10000 for the temple's construction in the village. In the FGD, the community also mentioned that people who have migrated to the cities for better earnings had contributed more significantly than rural households.

On the contrary, it was observed that a few households still do not have access to toilets and defecate in the open. They do not have sufficient money to construct the toilet, and most households have constructed it with the support of an incentive amount disbursed under SBM(G). Thus, the community collectively mobilised an substantial amount of money to construct a temple in the village. However, it contrastingly reflected community's lower priority and willingness to construct and use the toilet. In Chenguta block of Medak district, it was observed that women took some time to participate in the PRA where they shared their tacit knowledge and experiences. Participation by children was unexpected and revealed that they are the most aware and well-informed community members. Children are working

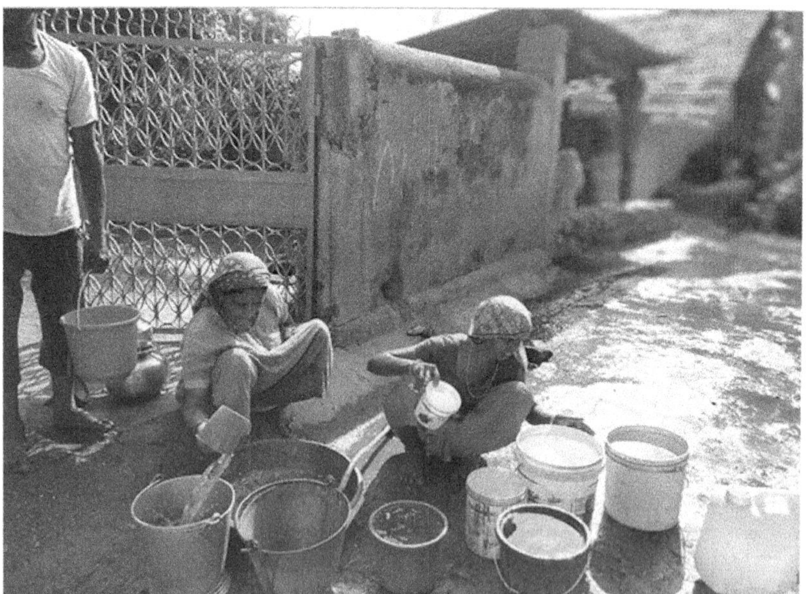

Figure 7.9 Water Storing for the Week.

Source: Author Deepa Gupta

as key informants and catalysts in the implementation process of SBM(G). They actively corrected and represented the physical resources, natural resources, demographical and geographical patterns, and also located the exact positions of the toilets constructed. Locating toilets in the houses was not enough to understand the villages' social realities. It was surprising that the community has marked the houses with differently abled persons. Differently abled persons in the community face various challenges of inappropriate sanitation structures, which are not user-friendly. Consequently, there is a pressing need for special provision and innovative toilet solutions to enhance the inclusivity of policy implementation at the grassroots level.

Community Behaviour Change

The construction target for SBM(G) implementation is for the rural households. These includes the households of daily wage or agricultural labourers who may not own land and face challenges in accessing to drinking water, toilets, and basic living conditions. Villages of Bihar are severely flood prone while the villages of Telangana grapple with the impacts of drought. Challenges faced by the community during the natural disasters led to the loss of income, poor access to basic amenities, and poor health and hygiene at the community level. In the Hasanpur block of Samastipur district, a few households not owning a land and temporarily residing on someone else's property. Some households lack separate spaces for essential household chores such as cooking, storing (see Figure 7.10), washing, and sleeping. Field observations revealed impoverished living conditions where residents had to contend with stagnant water or drains within temporary dwellings. For such households, access to exclusive sanitation facilities remains a distant aspiration. Field observations and discussions stated that the Sarairanjan block in the Samastipur district possesses better awareness regarding sanitation programmes than the Hasanpur block.

The primary factors contributing to better awareness were political will, involvement of district administration, access to information, and community participation. Consequently, the individual households in the rural villages became the focal point of the programme implementation. The programme required varied strategies to address the needs of the target households. Initiatives like Nukkad Natak, workshops, training, and awareness campaigns facilitated community mobilisation, participation, and awareness creation. During the visit, it was observed that some male members remained resistant to using the toilet and continued to practice open defecation. Older women faced challenges in abandoning the age-old practices of open defecation and adapting to the new behaviour of using the toilet. Non-adherence to toilet usage posed a significant concern. Therefore, necessitating the targeted social behaviour change communication strategy to address the specific needs of target group. It has been observed that Social Behaviour Change and Communication (SBCC) strategies were predominantly focused on shaping the behaviour of children and young women, overlooking the behavioural concerns of on male and older adults within household. Better health and hygiene

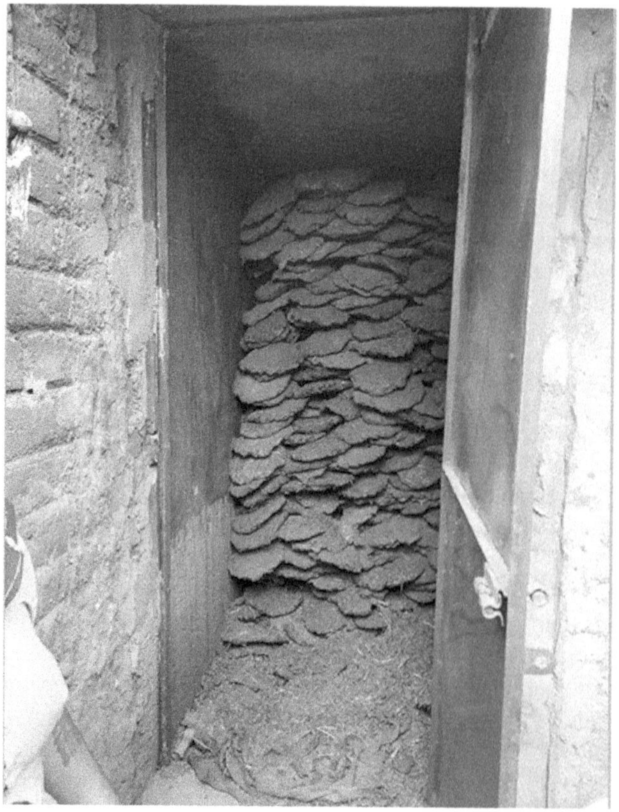

Figure 7.10 Toilet Used for Storage.

Source: Author Deepa Gupta

among children, adolescent girls, and young women are crucial, neglecting the behavioural concerns among male and older adults in the community creates substantial obstacles to achieving the goal of an open defecation-free country.

In Rampur village of Samastipur district, it was revealed that the delay in disbursement of sanitation incentives to individual households discouraged them from using and improving the sanitation structure. Women in the meeting stated that 'we are concerned about our personal and social well-being, but sanitation in the household is not everyone's priority. Though we face many challenges due to poor sanitation, other priority needs are seizing most of the resources and attention.' Further probing revealed that food security, owning a house, better education, entertainment, and access to better health services are significant household concerns. The sanitation initiatives and campaigns are focused on the right to dignity and better health and hygiene for all. Thus, the rural poor might not comprehend the relationship between poor sanitation and poor health. However, the policymaker needs more focus on understanding the challenges of males, older adults, and differently abled persons in the community.

During the FGD with women, it was reported that the school-going children have developed a habit of using toilets, thanks to training in handwashing and toilet use. During the informal discussions, children mentioned that they have appointed monitors among themselves, such as Bal Mantri , at the school to oversee their peers' adherence to proper sanitation practices. Consequently, they play a crucial role as vital information carriers to households and actively participate in fostering change. Further, it was reported that a large family with a twin pit toilet facility is somewhat hesitant about using the toilet due to the perception that the pit will fill up quickly. Consequently, only young newly wed women and children use the toilet, and others prefer to go for open defecation. Also, if the toilet is occupied, the other household members prefer to go for open defecation. Beyond these behavioural concerns, social myths are prevalent in the community and negatively influence the desired behaviour of using the toilet. It is a common belief across villages that constructing and using toilets within the dwelling may pollute the house's aura especially since worship and cooking occur in the same place. The community has also responded that it may also pollute groundwater quality if they construct the toilet near water sources.

Community behaviour and attitude towards cleaning and maintaining toilets is significant aspects of social behaviour change communication. During the discussion, members mentioned that they clean their houses but do not want to clean the toilet and dump the garbage on the roadside or at a common dumping space. In Medak, the Panchayat has addressed this concern by appointing a cleaner to perform weekly cleaning of individual toilets. In Samastipur, the community has also raised this concern that the administration should either appoint a cleaner or provide regular services to clean the household's toilet. Moreover, in Dahod, the community has mentioned that they face challenges cleaning and maintaining the toilet due to the severe water scarcity problem. Thus, the SBCC approach needs to emphasise the construction and usage of toilets and the ownership and responsibility for their regular cleaning and maintenance.

In Telangana, the households have been provided with two separate dustbins to segregate dry and wet waste. These bins are intended to be collected and disposed of at the waste treatment plant. The Panchayat took this initiative to change behaviour within the community regarding waste segregation at the household level. However, the choice of dustbins proved to be inappropriate, as they were reticulated and thus unsuitable for segregate the wet waste.

In Vikarabad, the unavailability of water was the primary concern for the low usage of the toilet. Conversely, in Samastipur, people refrained from using toilets due to the perception that the pit would fill up quickly, necessitating the laborious task of emptying it. Members also expressed their discomfort with the toilet structure, citing feelings of suffocation and darkness. Thus, these physical discomfort act as a barrier to embracing the recommended behavior. In various villages, community responses indicated a common practice of washing hands with soil and soap. If soap was unavailable, individuals did not hesitate to wash their hands with soil.

On the contrary, only a few households had access to soap near the water source during the household visit. It has also been observed that households use the toilet for other purposes, such as bathing, cleaning, and storing goods. In some cases, they have covered the toilet pan with a stone slab so no one can use it. Therefore, it is imperative to reevaluate strategies and address the diverse needs of different target groups to instigate behavioural change and bring behavioural change at both the individual and community levels. For example, one needs to investigate the reasons for not using toilets, debunk myths and norms associated with toilet usage, access and availability of toilets in public spaces, and identify challenges posed by existing toilet structures.

Physical Realities of WASH

The physical realities of villages relatively differ in terms of availability and accessibility to sanitation facilities. It includes the challenges related to water, sanitation, and hygiene. The difference in geographical and demographical patterns could be critical for disparities and physical realities for accessing water, sanitation, and hygiene facilities. Field visits to the selected villages suggest that perception, awareness, and socio-economic realities also played a vital role in shaping physical realities at the grassroots. Water availability in the Dahod district was identified as most challenging among all the districts, while water quality was subpar in the Samastipur district. In Samastipur, households predominantly relied on bottled water for drinking despite having easy access to hand pumps. The primary concern for the shift to bottled water was the high arsenic in the groundwater, negatively affecting community health.

On the contrary, Mission Bhagiratha has been successfully implemented in Telangana villages, yet the community continues to prefer bottled water for drinking purposes. Though the households have better access to water in Telangana through Mission Bhagiratha, households primarily utilised piped water supply for cleaning, bathing, and other household chores. In Bihar, most households owned hand pumps or have access to community hand pumps for water use. On the contrary, Gujarat villages still face the unavailability and inaccessibility of quality water. It has been observed that the best-performing districts and blocks have better access to water, sanitation, and hygiene. Dahod, as a least-performing district, faces severe challenges due to dependency on the unprotected water source for all the water use compared to other districts. Poor access to water is an essential factor negatively influencing sanitation usage. Residents have constructed a small one foot water tank to store drinking water for at least ten days (see Figure 7.9), as they are getting a piped water supply for a maximum of twice a month.

Furthermore, the dependence on the unprotected water source for various household chores is substantial. Implementing Mission Bhagiratha in Telangana villages has achieved the remarkable milestone of providing better access to water at the dwelling. The scheme advocates for individual piped water connections to all the villages' households. Though the scheme has benefitted the many in the village, certain segments, particularly lower caste hamlets, continue to face deprivation from its advantages. The villages have also observed conflicts over water connections among the community and government officials. The community was raising concerns about delays in water connection to the dwelling. In response, the officials mentioned that the delay was due to the lack of available funds. In Lingampally, the community mentioned that they used to get the water supply twice a day, but now it is not the case, and there are days when there is no supply. The community in Lingampally was paying Rs. 20 per month for two hours of water supply in the morning, while in Wadiyaram, they were paying Rs. 40 per month. In Rampur and Sarai Ranjan, the community purchased 20 litres of water bottles for Rs. 20 per bottle for drinking. In Allapur, the community is dependent on public water tanks for water supply as a pipeline to the dwelling has been laid, but the supply has not started yet. In the case of Malkapur and Konaipally, the households have access to the piped water supply. However, they prefer to buy water through water vending machines installed in the villages for drinking. Thus, they have been provided with a water ATM card to purchase water through the water vending machine. They were supposed to recharge that card and might swipe this to the machine whenever they needed to buy water. So, they used to purchase water at Rs. 5 per 20 litres of water. Therefore, the inadequate access to water in the village remains a significant cause, affecting the low usage of toilets.

The community also believed that constructing toilets near the water source or dwelling might degrade the water quality and pollute the locality. Therefore, also fear that it may cause an epidemic. The majority of the households in Bihar have constructed the septic tank instead of the twin pit. Demand for a twin pit latrine was deficient in the community despite its low cost. The community has responded that they prefer at least a 10- to 12-feet-deep septic tank instead of a 3-feet-deep twin pit. The reason behind the preference for a septic tank over a twin pit is that the household, especially the old members, does not want to fill it quickly and wants to avoid the associated burden of pit emptying. Moreover, the lower preference for soak pit toilets is attributed to the lack of proper space, limited awareness of the benefits of twin pit design, and the threat to degradation of groundwater quality. The community has also revealed that the current structure of toilets does not meet the needs of –differently abled persons. The number of toilets constructed, access to the toilet, awareness of SBM, and toilet usage were high in the best-performing districts compared to the least-performing ones. District administration in Sitamarhi district has developed the hamlet of scheduled caste as the model hamlet for sanitation. Individual toilets for the households have been constructed, and incentives were disbursed to the households on a priority basis. On the contrary, the community's use of the toilets was put on hold, and they were advised to use it after the inauguration ceremony planned by the district administration and local vital persons, i.e., PRI members, contractors, etc. The incident was a little awful as this delay caused some dissatisfaction within the community, as they had been eagerly awaiting the opportunity to use the newly constructed toilets for more than two weeks.

On the other hand, in Dahod, the households are demographically scattered, and the agricultural fields surround the village. The households may not recognise the necessity for toilets as they have ample space for open defecation. The challenge of community mobilisation has contributed to the lack of awareness in the Dahod district. In Sabarkantha, most of the toilets in the household were locked as the families migrated to the cities for better employment opportunities. The households were observed using toilets for other household chores like bathing, washing, cleaning, storing fodder or water, etc., both in Telangana and Bihar. Seasonal migration and discomfort with the existing physical structure were a few reasons for the household's low demand for twin pit toilets. Across the villages, it has been observed that the construction of toilets appeared to be a low priority.

Despite owning houses, households have not incorporated toilet construction into their building plan. Wadiyaram has been declared Open Defecation Free (ODF), but most twin pits were incomplete and damaged. Lower caste households in Wadiyaram were opting for open defecation instead of using the toilets, citing the main reason as the underfurnished and damaged structures (see Figure 7.11). Telangana was the only state where the community members mentioned that the toilet was constructed converging with other schemes, such as NREGA. Existing norms and beliefs associated with the toilet have also influenced its usage in the household.

Community in Telangana villages believed that households with pregnant women should not construct a toilet. In Bihar, pollution and purity were prevalent; thus, the community did not prefer building toilets within the dwelling. Also, in the villages of Bihar, women are not allowed to take water for open defecation. If a woman did so, it was seen as an act of shamelessness, inviting potential mishaps. However, they wash and clean themselves after returning home from open defecation. Women are not supposed to take water to the field during menstruation, which is unhygienic and troublesome. These gendered norms highlight societal biases and irrationality, indicating a low priority and sensitivity towards women's health and hygiene.

Most households do not have access to separate bathing spaces and usually bathe near the primary water source or shared space in the dwelling. Similarly, members wash their hands after using toilets or general cleaning near the primary water source. Moreover, in Telangana, the community members mentioned that they only wash their hands inside the toilets, which was not the case in Bihar and Gujarat. Sometimes they use soap or wash their hands with ash or soil. The poor drainage system in the villages of Hasanpur and Dahod was critical for community hygiene, while in Malkapur, an uncovered drain with waste collection chambers led to issues like mosquitoes, flies, insects, and foul smells in the village.

Across all the study areas, the villages lack proper arrangements for solid-liquid waste management, leading villagers to dispose of garbage in familiar dumping places. Furthermore, poor community mobilisation and participation, limited awareness, low priority to construct toilets, low usage of toilets, no separate bathing and washing space, poor water quality, water unavailability, poor drainage system, and lack of solid-liquid waste management system were critical reasons for poor sanitation status of the village. Furthermore, political will, active local administration, involvement of civil society organisations, participation of women, children, and youths, inclusive approach to communication, and timely disbursement of funds played a vital role in promoting the construction and usage of a sanitation facility at the community and household levels.

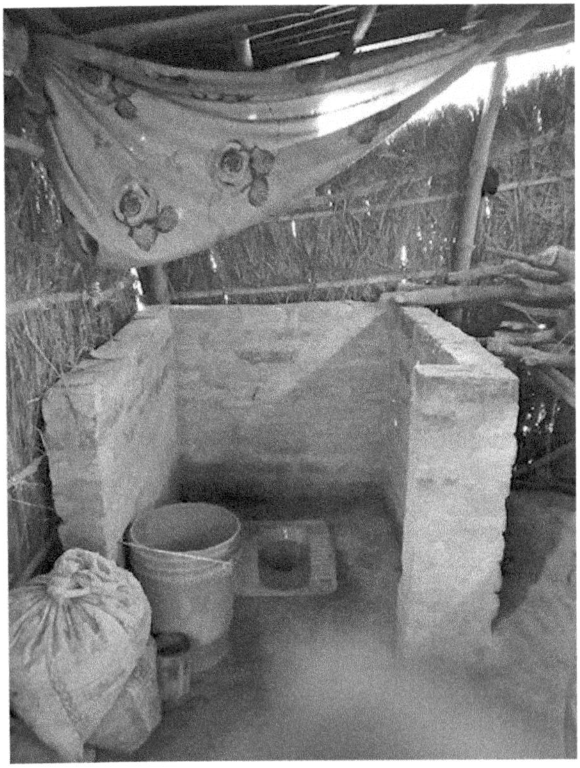

Figure 7.11 Use of Toilet.

Source: Author Deepa Gupta

Conclusion

The chapter highlighted the role of public and community institutions in sanitation behaviour and the physical realities of water, sanitation, and hygiene at the grassroots. The exploratory study suggests that the role of local bodies and administration differs even in the identical institutional set-up. The best-performing districts demonstrate a more substantial involvement of district administration at every stage of planning, implementation, and monitoring of sanitation programs. However, at the same time, it has also been investigated that better engagement of district and local administration may lead to successful short-term outcomes, it may not guarantee a sustainable approach to implementing public schemes. The best-performing districts passionately invested in achieving all the set targets of SBM(G) in the districts; on the other hand, the least-performing ones were inconsistent, less involved, and less attentive to achieving sanitation targets. It has also been observed that the government officials have less priority in visiting demographically challenged regions and thus shifted the whole focus of implementing SBM(G) to the best-connected districts. Guidelines of SBM(G) suggest the convergence of the programme with small collectives such as SHGs, Cluster Level Federations, and government schemes such as MGNREGA and NRLM. It has the potential to create livelihoods for the rural poor and capacity building and to empower existing institutional networks. However, the convergence of programmes with other schemes and institutions has diverse challenges too. This includes delays in fund disbursement, political influence, caste-based politics, and transfer of incentives in multiple instalments.

Small collectives and external funding also play a crucial role in sustaining the behaviour change. Community institutions have been instrumental in facilitating community mobilisation, demand generation for toilet construction, usage of toilets, and waste segregation in the household. Women and youth groups have played a vital role in implementing SBM(G). In the initial stage, rural households needed monetary support and thus took loans from small collectives. Therefore, SHG members have taken a loan to construct the toilet from the SHAN fund from SHGs and Village Organizations. In certain districts, incentives were disbursed in more than two instalments with some provided upon the completion of toilet construction. Morning vigilance, whistle-blowing, meetings, training, workshops, *Tatti par Matti*, Nukkad Natak, door-to-door visits, rallies, wall paintings, billboards, oath taking for toilet use (see Figure 7.7), and the appointment of Swacchatagrahi, etc. were a few initiatives taken to create awareness and disseminate information to stop open defecation.

The unexpected participation by children revealed that they are the most aware and well-informed community members. Children are working as key informants and catalysts in the implementation process of SBM(G). The participation of the community in sanitation activities and campaigns depends on various dynamics such as access to public institutions, knowledge and information, social networks, age, caste, gender, and social norms. The Swacchatagrahi facilitated the toilet demand to the Panchayat and smoothly disbursed incentives to the households.

Most households in the community have constructed toilets outside the dwelling, and many refrain from using them due to the prevailing social norms. It is a common belief across villages that constructing and using toilets within the dwelling may pollute the house's aura where worship and cooking occur. Additionally, it may also degrade groundwater quality. A large family with a twin pit toilet facility remains skeptical about using the toilet, fearing that it might fill up quickly. Households, even though they own the house, have not planned to construct a toilet during the construction of the house. The SBCC approach needs to focus on ownership of toilets by the household to construct and use them and clean and maintain them. It is critical to revisit the strategies to address the needs of different target groups, perceptions of not using toilets, myths, and norms associated with not using toilets.

The community exhibited a lack of demand for twin pit latrines despite their affordability. The reason behind the preference for a septic tank over a twin pit, especially among older members, is the pit filling up quickly and the associated hassle of emptying it. Additionally, the lower preference for soak pit toilets was due to lack of proper space, low awareness of the benefits of twin pit design, and threat to degradation of groundwater quality. The households used toilets for other household chores like bathing, washing, cleaning, storing fodder or water, etc. The inadequate access to water in the village poses a significant challenge, leading to limited toilet usage. Moreover, most households lack separate bathing spaces, often resorting to bathing near the primary water source or shared spaces within the dwelling.

Low priority and willingness to construct and use toilets reflect the community's attitude and perception. People fear social sanctions or penalties and have changed their place and timings for open defecation even after constructing the toilet. Male members generally disapprove of imposing penalties for open defecation. On the other hand, the women groups mentioned that the felicitation for adopting best sanitation practices might motivate other households in the locality to adopt advocated behaviour (see Figure 7.4). Notably, resistance to toilet usage persists among some male members, while older women find it challenging to forsake the traditional practice of open defecation. It has been observed that SBCC strategies were more focused on addressing the behaviour of children and young women and lacked emphasis on male and older adults in the household.

Better health and hygiene among children, adolescent girls, and young women are crucial, yet overlooking the behavioural concerns among male and older adults in the community creates substantial obstacles to achieving the objective of an open defecation-free country. Differently abled persons in the community face various challenges of inappropriate sanitation structures, i.e., they are not user friendly. Consequently, there is an urgent need for special provision and a range of innovative toilet solutions to ensure the policy implementation at the grassroots.

However, the policymaker needs more focus on understanding the challenges of males, older adults, and differently abled persons in the community. Political will, active local administration, involvement of civil society organisations, participation of women, children, and youths, inclusive approach to communication, and timely disbursement of funds played a vital role in promoting the construction and usage of a sanitation facility at the community and household levels. Furthermore, poor community mobilisation and participation, less awareness, low priority to construct toilets, low usage of toilets, no separate bathing and washing space, poor quality of water, unavailability of water, poor drainage system, and lack of solid-liquid waste management system were critical reasons for poor sanitation status of the village.

8 Discussion and Policy Implications

Access to water and sanitation for all is one of the Sustainable Development Goals (SDG-6) set by the United Nations. Access to sanitation has immense importance for good physical and mental health. Lack of sanitation spreads infectious diseases and can have an overall negative impact on the development of a nation. A recent study in India reveals that health-related net benefits of rural sanitation intervention are to the tune of USD 13 and USD 10 per person per year, and benefit-cost ratios are 2.5 and 5 in Karnataka and Uttar Pradesh, respectively (Weis et al., 2019). Understanding the importance of sanitation, the prime minister of India, Shri Narendra Modi, launched the Swachh Bharat Mission (SBM), a public sanitation programme, in October 2014 to make India open defecation free by October 2019. However, this is not the first sanitation programme in India. There is a long history of public intervention in sanitation in the country.

This book attempts to delineate and analyse the principal drivers (social, cultural, physical, and behavioural) that motivate people to stop open defecation and use the toilet. What is novel about this book is that it discusses access to sanitation in the overall context of access to other essential services and social and cultural norms. Only a handful of studies have considered social norms and values. The normative aspects of sanitation behaviour are important as open defecation may be an expected and widely accepted behaviour deeply rooted in the local culture. This book fills this gap by analysing people's attitudes towards sanitation.

Public Sanitation Programme in India

As mentioned in the previous chapters, the Central Rural Sanitation Programme (CRSP) was launched in 1986 by the Ministry of Rural Development. This programme was launched after the government realised that the benefits of the rural water supply programme could not be fully realised unless the sanitary aspects of water and the issue of sanitation were addressed together. This programme was highly subsidised. The programme provided a 100% subsidy for the construction of sanitary toilets for scheduled castes, scheduled tribes, and landless labourers. Moreover, the programme was supply driven and emphasised a single construction model.

Rural sanitation strategy changed in the IXth Plan from a high-subsidy to a low-subsidy regime, with greater household involvement, choice of technology

DOI: 10.4324/9781032726267-8

according to customer preference, stress on software, etc. The programme was revised based on the recommendations of the National Seminar on Rural Sanitation in 1992. A new programme was launched as the Total Sanitation Campaign (TSC) in 1999, following a community-led, people-centric, and 'demand-driven' approach. It is based on the successful model of the Midnapur district of West Bengal, called the 'Midnapur Model'. The programme emphasises information, education, and communication (IEC) for demand generation for sanitation facilities. In addition, to meet the demand for sanitation facilities, alternative delivery mechanisms in the form of production centres and Rural Sanitary Marts (RSMs) were set up (GOI, 2001, 2004).

TSC was a Centrally Sponsored Scheme (CSS). The state government must provide matching contributions under the Minimum Needs Programme (MNP). Financial support in the form of a 20% subsidy was given to construct individual household toilets for those below the poverty line (BPL). Financial assistance was also provided to government rural schools, Anganwadis, and Balwadi centres for toilet construction, emphasising separate toilets for girls in all co-educational schools. Community Sanitary Complexes for women in villages were constructed where land was available, and the community was ready to own, operate, and maintain such complexes.

In October 2014, the Swachh Bharat Mission (SBM) was launched by the government, and by October 2019, India was declared 'open-defecation free' (ODF). Under this programme, the beneficiaries were provided with a subsidy of Rs. 12000 for the construction of twin pit toilets. Under this programme, more than 169 million household toilets were constructed. Despite such monumental achievement, ODF sustainability, meaning the elimination of open defecation, is a matter of concern (Mehta, 2018). According to the SBM programme, the local administrative system must engage with the ODF village for nine months after the ODF declaration. The mission has moved towards the Phase-II of SBM as ODF Plus, whereby focus has been given to solid and liquid waste management to sustain open defecation-free behaviour. It is argued that ODF Plus activities are critical for ensuring ODF sustainability. This phase will reinforce ODF behaviour and focus on the safe management of solid and liquid waste in villages.

Study of Three States

The empirical investigation of the study has been conducted in three different states of India: Bihar, Gujarat, and Telangana. According to the Ministry of Culture, Government of India, Bihar is in the North Central Culture Zone, Gujarat is in the West Culture Zone, and Telangana is in the South Culture Zone. In 2018, when the study was initiated, the access to sanitation was lowest in Bihar, medium in Telangana, and highest in Gujarat. To make the data representative of these states, the best- and worst-performing districts and blocks were selected to make the sample representative. We surveyed 1252 sample households with the help of a pre-designed questionnaire in these three states taken together. The household members, especially the household heads, were the survey respondents. To understand the sanitation behaviour of rural households in depth, a qualitative study was conducted through in-depth structured and unstructured interviews. The Zaltman Metaphor Elicitation Technique (Z-MET) and Participatory Rural Appraisal (PRA) were conducted to understand the households' perspective of sanitation, perception of their social environment, and availability of social infrastructure and resources.

The sample households' general characteristics leave many implications for sanitation behaviour. The number of members per household was large. On average, there were six members per household. Hence, if only one toilet is built in the household, it may be difficult for every member to use it appropriately, especially in larger households. We found that households are backward regarding their education and social identity, such as caste. Around 21% of males and 35% of females are illiterate. In the overall sample, 38% belong to the scheduled caste, and 20% belong to the scheduled tribe.

The economic status of the households also matters in sanitation behaviour. The economic condition of households appears to be the best in Gujarat and worst in Bihar. There are wide variations across districts of the states. The economic backwardness of households is likely to have a negative impact on the adoption of toilets. The expenditure pattern of households, which depicts their economic condition and expenditure priority, varied across states. The households mainly spent on necessities like food, medicine, and education. It implies that they did not have many surplus resources.

The occupation of households determines their professional and social exposure. More exposure outside the traditional employment is likely to encourage behaviour change in sanitation. We observe that around 60% of households were agricultural self-employed, while around 20% were regular wage or salary earners. The primary living condition of the households was poor. Almost half of the dwellings had their floor and wall made of *Kaccha* materials, while most had roofs made of *Pucca*. Half of the households did not have access to the bathroom. Poor living conditions may deter households from constructing toilets as they may adopt toilets when overall living conditions improve. By June–September 2018, during the survey, around one-third of the sample households did not have access to a toilet. The lack of access was higher in some areas than in others in the same state. The use of toilets was much higher for Muslims and Christians than for Hindus. Interestingly, access to a toilet was higher for upper castes, but the use of the toilet by all members of households was lower for them. There were wide variations in access to sanitation within the state. In some districts such as Samastipur and Dahod, more than half of households had no toilet access.

The demographic composition of the household influences the use of toilets. If the number of household members is higher, the chance of using the toilet reduces for males above 15 years. A larger family size also reduces the chances of using the toilet by all the members. Furthermore, if the percentage of females in a household increases, males above 15 years are less likely to use the toilet; these results imply that with as many members in a household, many members find the toilets occupied during the prime time of their use. Females prioritise males using the toilet while males choose open defecation to avoid waiting. Education does not have any statistically significant impact on toilet access. But if the highest level of education of female members of households is 10th standard (or ten years of schooling), then female adults and children are more likely to use the toilet. Access to other essential services matters for the access and use of a toilet. Access to piped water supply in the dwelling, access to drinking water, and access to a bathroom for the household's exclusive use improve both access and use of a toilet. Hence, the general living standard of households has implications for access to and use of a toilet. Social norms may have implications for toilet use.

In many cases, social norms of purity hindered the construction of toilets within the dwelling. Access to the toilet was better for the higher economic class, but the use of a toilet by all members was best in the lowest economic class. A household was more likely to have access to a toilet if its monthly consumption expenditure (a proxy for income) was higher. Those who had not constructed toilets could not do so due to financial constraints. Toilet use by males and females over 15 years of age (not all family members) was likely higher if they spent more on durable goods and entertainment. People spend more on durable goods and entertainment when they have surplus resources. Hence, adults are more likely to use the toilet when they have surplus resources. It may be because people want a better living standard with more availability of resources. Toilet use is a different means of achieving a better living standard.

Swachh Bharat Mission (SBM) left a lot to be desired. SBM promoted pit toilets, but only 12% of households had them. Our further studies reveal that people were hesitant to use pit toilets because they feared they would get filled quickly. It is best indicated by the fact that Dahod, where the pit toilet was most prevalent, had the highest percentage of households not using the toilet. The overall sanitation and public health conditions of the villages were also poor. Besides lack of sanitation, many households reported problems like stomach upset, fever, etc. Around 90% of households suffered from the nuisance of mosquitoes and flies. It implies that overall public health conditions in the villages were poor.

Convenience and privacy have appeared to be the two most important factors for toilet construction. The regression analysis suggests that female-headed households are more likely to have access to the toilet. Furthermore, if the percentage of female members in the households is higher, then it is less likely for males below 15 years of age to use the toilet. Due to the importance of privacy and safety, female members prioritise toilet use. Alongside, potential health benefits were one of the significant reasons for toilet construction. However, there are concerns as people reported that they were forced or coerced by officials or leaders to construct a toilet. It was reported by only a few households but needed to be resisted for the programme's success. The sanitation programme should be self-driven. Essentially it holds in survey villages. Most of the toilet constructions were influenced by self or spouse. We did not observe any significant role of health or social workers in influencing people for behavioural change.

There was sufficient awareness about SBM in the survey villages. People knew about SBM through TV and radio broadcasting, meetings, and public functions.

We observed that awareness about SBM reduced the chances of open defecation by 10%. Again, external influence and force were behind people attending meetings. Despite knowledge about SBM, many were not convinced about problems of open defecation and instead perceived it as beneficial. A substantial proportion of people believed that open defecation did not threaten privacy. People considered open defecation an opportunity to discuss important matters. Despite general ignorance, there was a substantial demand for good-quality toilets with doors and other safety measures. Many households consider the toilet more critical than mobile phones and bicycles. Community participation was essential for the overall change in sanitation behaviour. The households were unable or unwilling to use the toilet for various reasons, which may be attributable to the design. The twin pit toilet promoted by SBM was unacceptable for most households. They feared that it would eventually contaminate groundwater. There were problems with cleaning the filled pits as well. They cannot afford flush toilets, and if the space inside the toilet is small, it discourages people from using the toilet. Small space is one of the characteristics of toilets built under SBM. Households that could afford added extra money to build flush toilets with septic tanks or large pits that would take a decade to fill.

Policy Implications

The lack of sanitation facilities for rural masses is not entirely due to low income but a host of other factors, including behavioural issues. The general living standard of people determines their preference for sanitation. People's preference for sanitation may trail behind the preference for several other essential amenities. On the other hand, social norms of purity may discourage households from constructing toilets inside or even within the premises. The avoidance of toilets may get exacerbated if the quality of construction is not up to the mark or the structure is inconvenient for use. The unavailability of sufficient water supply may make the situation worse. The implementation mechanism is not always efficient. Information, education, and communication (IEC) are either inadequate or ineffective in generating demand for sanitation. An institutional mechanism with a proper incentive structure to discourage open defecation is mostly not in place. The sanitation policies should be able to address these issues.

Economic Development

Income along with higher expenditure on durable goods impacts the uptake of sanitation. Sanitation programme is more likely to succeed in regions where employment and income generation programmes are delivered efficiently. An aspirational household with increasing income and living standards is likelier to build and use the toilet. Hence, sanitation programmes should converge with other employment generation or livelihood programmes.

In this context, it is crucial to converge sanitation programmes with other economic development programmes, including access to essential services. Pradhan Mantri Awaas Yojana-Gramin (PMAY-G) may be a case. In this programme, monetary support is provided to construct the house. Within the ambit of the programme, the beneficiaries are also employed under Mahatma Gandhi National Rural Employment Guarantee Scheme (MGNREGS) and given Rs. 12000 for toilet construction under SBM. However, such an integrated approach should include water supply to households. There should be support such as direct subsidies or subsidised loans to construct bathrooms for already built houses. It is because bathrooms are essential for toilet use. The income of households should be enhanced in the same villages through MGNREGS or the National Rural Livelihood Mission (NRLM). The Self-Help Groups (SHGs) created under NRLM can also be motivated for toilet use. An integrated approach can only make behaviour change in sanitation. However, without an increase in the agricultural income and wages for agricultural workers, it will be nearly impossible to maintain the toilets in the long run.

Dealing with Social Norms

Open defecation practised in a locality may be reinforced because of collective behaviour. To deal with collective behaviour, it is essential to understand its nature. Bicchieri's (2016) work on collective behaviour may be considered. People may prefer to follow a collective behaviour irrespective of what others do. This type of collective behaviour is ascribed as collective custom.

On the other hand, people may display specific behaviour by only following others or by observing others. There could be two types of situations while following others. A person may follow others as they get motivated by others. This type of collective behaviour can be ascribed as descriptive norms. In another situation, a person may follow others as others expect the person to follow the behaviour. In the latter situation, the behaviour is institutionalised, and there are penalties for not following such behaviour. This type of collective behaviour is the social norm.

The influence of collective behaviour on individuals depends on their interconnectedness. De et al. (2021) found that interpersonal interactions about sanitation may have varied spread and nature across societies and cultures. It may be broad in some cultures and smaller or fragmented in others. The nature of connections may also be different: in some cultures, it may be more reciprocal, and in others, it may be less. An understanding of social networks may provide an understanding of the intervention strategy.

The nature of intervention would be different when the collective behaviour is a custom vis-à-vis descriptive or social norms. If it is a custom, people follow a collective behaviour, say open defecation, as they find it the best strategy. They would do so if they could not appreciate the importance of the toilet. Health and social workers may play an essential role in this context. A financial constraint may be one of the reasons for open defecation. Hence, a strategy of IEC and public sanitation programmes may be helpful. Gupta et al. (2016) argued that it is essential to confront notions of purity and pollution and teach people about the germ theory of disease. The quality of toilets developed under the sanitation programme matters significantly. De et al. (2021) found that the personal belief that the toilet provides safety and convenience was prevalent, but the belief varied across cultures. Our study also observed the same. Hence, with economic support and IEC, motivating people to construct and use the toilet is possible. If personal normative beliefs are high, it is possible to motivate toilet use even if it is socially sanctioned. De et al. (2021) observed that a substantial proportion of households constructed toilets despite shaming by neighbours for toilet construction.

In case collective behaviour such as open defecation is influenced by observing others, social and political leaders must influence people to change their behaviour. Each one should influence others to change their behaviour. It is in addition to the role played by health and social workers, including IEC and the subsidised government sanitation programme, which provide good-quality toilets. The role of social and political leaders is even more crucial if the collective behaviour is a social norm rather than a descriptive norm. Since social norms are institutionalised, the social and political leaders may not want any behaviour change. They may not be motivated or convinced. In such a situation, the programme implementers must meet and convince every leader or influencer of the locality. Intervention at the contact nodes in the villages should be considered a general behaviour change strategy.

Change in sanitation behaviour is a collective activity. If a few community members continue to defecate in the open, it may discourage and disincentivise others to change their behaviour. It may be helpful to develop informal norms for behavioural change. Mutual monitoring against open defecation could be a way to tackle the problem of open defecation. Social sanctions or fines for open defecation may encourage toilet use. It has been observed by De et al. (2021) that people were taunted, mocked, and even driven away from fields for open defecation. People want social or financial sanctions to contain open defecation in areas where personal normative beliefs primarily drive sanitation behaviour. However, such sanctions should not be indecent, burdensome, and coercive. The penalty for open defecation should be optimum and imposed in a graduated manner, as detailed by Ostrom (1990). It should be phased out once a large proportion of people stop open defecation.

In this context, community-led total sanitation (CLTS) is worth mentioning. It is an approach to sanitation intervention where instead of incentivising people through subsidy, the intervention process ignites a collective sense of disgust and shame among the community members (Kar & Chambers, 2008). One of the essential elements in the process is triggering, where the intervention triggers self-realisation among community members that they need to change their satiation behaviour. In the post-triggering stage, community action is ensured through natural leaders in the intervention process. Follow-up actions are taken to construct and use toilets, and punishment or penalty is imposed for open defecation. Research in Ghana reveals that if people strongly identify with their social group, their sense of belongingness with the group is high, and their group identity is an integral part of their self-image. Behaviour change through CLTS is very effective (Hater et al., 2019). This is because people want to be accepted and approved by the group. TSC was based on the community-led total sanitation (CLTS) programme that had tasted success in Bangladesh and was spread across with the support of several international donor organisations, including the World Bank. CLTS was adopted in 59 countries worldwide and incorporated many changes based on the local context. However, the fundamental principles were the same, which included leveraging emotional aspects such as shame, pride, fear, and dignity for community mobilisation and using Participatory Rural Appraisal (PRA) techniques like transect walks to sensitise communities to the problems of open defecation (Zuin et al., 2019).

The intervention policy for behavioural change in sanitation should nudge people to adopt an improved behaviour. Thaler and Sunstein (2008) describe nudging for behaviour change vividly. The initiatives that cost households in the short run but yield benefits in the long run and are uncertain are good for nudging. On the one hand, toilet use may have immediate financial and social (negative) implications. On the other hand, people are habituated to open defecation. Public health benefits and benefits of higher living standards and social status can only be realised in the long run. Public information about gradual behaviour change in society may be disseminated to nudge sanitation behaviour. It would give the impression that it is now an accepted practice and that not using the toilet is odd. Accepting toilet use as a better quality of life would reduce the risk of social sanctions for toilet use.

Quality of Sanitation

The design of the toilets should be moderated with multiple options to meet people's expectations. The designs should commeasure with the aspiration of the households. People consider the toilet as a mark of better living standards. Along with the design, the construction material should be upgraded. The toilets should be provided with a provision for water supply. In this regard, the 'Comprehensive Water Supply & Sanitation' project of Gram Vikas, an NGO, is worth studying. Toilets and bathing rooms (with RCC roof) with round-the-clock water supply to each toilet and kitchen for rural households in Odisha provide pathways to improve the living standards of households. This approach is in contrast to the construction of only toilets under different government sanitation programmes. Thus, it improves the overall quality of sanitation in poor households.

The twin pit toilet promoted by SBM is one major hindrance to toilet use. There is a fear of groundwater contamination by faecal matters deposited in the toilet pits. These fears are widespread and are not unfounded. In a study in the areas that sit on the top of hard rocks in India, it was observed that the soak pit toilets contaminate 100-metre-deep well water through fractures and fissures (Bhallamudi et al., 2019). The contamination is reduced if septic tanks replace soak pit toilets.

The design of the toilet also has implications. One main reason for not constructing a toilet is the twin pits of around three feet each, which are perceived to be small and would get filled very soon. Households perceive the removal of sludge from filled pits as problematic. In this context, Gupta et al. (2016) suggested emptying a pit is not manual scavenging. Having more than one option with varying design and construction materials is also necessary. The designs should have options for a twin pit on the one hand and a septic tank on the other hand.

It is recommended that there be options for larger pit sizes to dissuade the fear of it getting filled quickly, and the toilet room or superstructure is perceived as narrow and inconvenient. People feel suffocated in the narrow and filthy (if not cleaned properly due to water unavailability) toilets. Hence, there should be multiple options for superstructure: narrow, medium, and large. As using the toilet is an aspiration that develops with increasing living standards, the general cleanliness of households and locality may impact demand for sanitation positively. The villagers, especially the youth, may devote a specific amount of time every day to general cleanliness. The villages should have facilities like collection and disposal of waste and drainage facilities. It is advisable to form groups to conduct and monitor these activities. These collective efforts would, in turn, ensure ODF sustainability.

Government Policy and Initiatives

Convergence of government policies should be the prime focus, as discussed earlier. The overall sanitation situation should be considered, and a strategy should be developed to improve it. A bathroom facility and water supply should be provided along with toilets. Overall cleanliness of the villages, including garbage disposal and drainage, should be integrated into the public sanitation programme. Employment and livelihood programmes should also be part of the integrated approach. The government programme should also consider constructing more than one toilet for larger households. A single toilet in an enormous household dissuades male members from using the toilet and encourages open defecation. If there is a higher percentage of female members in a household, it is also advisable to have more than one toilet, especially in larger households. It is common in villages for more than one family to reside in a single household or within the same premises. In such households, the number of toilets should equal the number of families residing in the household.

The implementation mechanism should be made more efficient in places where payment delays are reported. Directly transferring the reimbursement amount to the bank accounts of beneficiaries is advisable. The villagers should be made more aware of the key persons, such as Swacchhagrahis, for better contact and quick processing of applications. Recruitment and appointment of Swacchhagrahis could be an important step in this direction. It would boost programme implementation and monitoring at the micro level.

Health and social workers should be more activated to motivate households for toilet construction and use. The health and social workers should play a pivotal role in ensuring that households use the toilet. ASHA workers can be trained to dispel misinformation and inform people how faecally transmitted infections inhibit growth and stunt children (Gupta et al., 2016). Households should be motivated and monitored even after the construction of toilets. Along with Swacchhagrahis, other health and social workers should be given incentives for conducting these activities. Dissemination of general health information by health workers can make households aspire to better health and give up open defecation.

The IEC activities may be strengthened. Our regression analysis suggests that having no awareness about SBM increases the chances of open defecation. Hence, general awareness about public sanitation programmes should be enhanced. Furthermore, government machinery at the village level should decide the mode of IEC effective in the region. Public functions such as street play or folk songs may be more effective in some locations.

On the other hand, in other locations, public meetings may be more effective in ushering behaviour change in sanitation. Government officials and political leaders should refrain from forcing or coercing people to attend these programmes. If it happens, it would be impossible to usher behaviour change. There should be monitoring from the upper levels of government that such incidents are not happening. Moreover, the work appraisal of the officers should be less dependent on physical achievements such as toilet construction and IEC activity conducted. It should be more oriented towards achieving the outcome, i.e., behavioural change.

Construction materials should be made available more quickly. The government should find ways to implement the programme at a lower cost using cheaper local materials. The district-level public health engineering departments may be entrusted with the job of research and development for using cheaper local materials for construction. Furthermore, cheaper chemicals for cleaning the toilets should be made available as the standard materials available in the market are costly. It would partially resolve the problems of foul smell and untidiness of toilets.

The SBM is a central government programme with construction targets. It is imperative that state-level government institutions also participate, especially in monitoring and implementation. State-level annual legislative reports should ensure better accountability and scrutiny (Sarkar & Bharat, 2021). The lack of accountability and scrutiny has led to the non-standard design of septic tanks for household toilets and less efficient excreta management (Chandana & Rao, 2021). The lack of enforcement of standards by governing bodies has led to this problem.

Overall, political will is one of the critical determinants of sanitation coverage. The variation in achievements across states may be partly accountable for it. However, the politicians should not make interventions at the household level. Politicians contacting the potential beneficiaries may put them under pressure. It may distort the process of demand generation for sanitation. Health and social workers should be entrusted with motivating people to construct and use toilets. However, politicians should put more effort into monitoring the activities of these workers. They should put more effort into IEC activities.

Women's Empowerment

Toilets are constructed and used primarily for privacy, safety, and convenience. Women are primary beneficiaries of toilet construction and use. According to O'Reilly (2016), without access to household toilets, women in low-income areas face three types of insecurity: (1) material lack due to not having toilet access, (2) risk of venturing out for open defecation, and (3) unstable and unsafe access if they access public toilet. Women's empowerment should have positive implications for toilet construction. Our study also reveals that women have a significant role in toilet construction and use. Female-headed households are more likely to have access to the toilet. Women may not be the decision-makers in other households, but they influence their spouses for toilet construction.

Women's influence in sanitation can be bolstered through overall improvement in women's agency. Women's agency determines their ability to make choices (Kabeer, 1999). Women's agency may improve through employment and income generation. It would be more effective if women were employed outside the traditional sectors or occupations (De, 2022). Women's agency may improve more when bargaining vertically in commercial engagements (Sifaki, 2019). Hence, women's work opportunities must improve in sectors that make them more empowered. Education would also enhance women's empowerment. Our regression analysis reveals that if the highest level of education for the females in the household is 10th standard (or ten years of education), then females of all ages are more likely to use the toilet.

Toilet construction and use may become more manageable if the intervention occurs through Self-Help Groups (SHGs) in the villages. Although SHGs are meant to provide small loans to rural women and develop economic activities, they may be helpful avenues for intervention in sanitation. SHGs empower women through exposure to the larger world and capacity building due to member engagement in group governance and income generation (Sanyal, 2009). The SHG women can usher behavioural change in their households and others.

Improved Targeting

Access to toilets is dependent on the income and social background of households. Our analysis suggests that people with higher consumption expenditure (a proxy for higher income) are more likely to use toilet and backward castes are more likely to go for open defecation. It calls for targeting lower-income households and backward castes. In two ways, targeting could be better: (1) More resources for IEC and more innovative approaches in areas dominated by tribal and backward castes. It should entail IEC material in the local language akin to local culture. (2) Subsidy for lower-income households should be increased so that they may be able to construct better-quality toilets.

Those not in deep poverty can contribute their resources to construct a better-quality toilet. It increases the chances of the use of the toilet. When impoverished people cannot contribute their own resources, government should provide more. For operational convenience, people under Antyodaya Anna Yojana (AAY), a section identified as the poorest, can be given a higher subsidy.

IEC activities should be strengthened in areas where migration is higher and households are headed by older people (more than 60 years). A case in point is the Sabarkantha district of Gujarat. The per capita monthly expenses (an indicator of economic well-being) are much higher in the Sabarkantha district. But public health measures such as street cleaning, garbage collection, water cleaning, and health check-ups are much less undertaken. Among households with access to a toilet in Sabarkantha, in 10% of households, all members do not use the toilet. Due to rural-urban migration, many villages in India are more inhabited by the elderly while the younger people live in towns or cities. The behaviour change in these villages is somewhat tricky. More intense and innovative IEC is required in these villages.

Overall, India has marched a long distance in making the country free from open defecation. Despite its monumental success, there are concerns regarding the ODF sustainability of the villages. The ODF Plus in SBM II may be helpful for overall sanitation and ODF sustainability. However, there is a need to reorient the approach to development intervention. Convergence of different government programmes is essential. The government must take the local community and intervene according to local conditions, particularly local networks of influence. The IEC programmes should be designed to sync with local culture and language. One crucial improvement area is the design of toilets and the quality of infrastructure. The community should also take responsibility by monitoring and imposing sanctions if needed. The intervention strategy may be channelled through women groups like SHGs. The poorest should be given higher support to build quality toilet infrastructure.

References

Agarwal, J., & Malhotra, N. K. (2005). An integrated model of attitude and affect: Theoretical foundation and an empirical investigation. *Journal of Business Research*, *58*(4), 483–493.

Alam, M. A., Richard, S. A., Fahim, S. M., Mahfuz, M., Nahar, B., Das, S., ... Ahmed, T. (2020). Impact of early-onset persistent stunting on cognitive development at 5 years of age: Results from a multi-country cohort study. *PLoS One*, *15*(1), e0227839.

Anca Christina Micu, J. T. (2010, June). Measurable emotions: Hoe television Ads really work. Patters of reactions to commercials can demonstrate advertising effectiveness. *Journal of Advertising Research*, 50(2), 137–153. DOI: 10.2501/S0021849910091300.

Andres, L., Briceño, B., Chase, C., & Echenique, J. A. (2017). Sanitation and externalities: Evidence from early childhood health in rural India. *Journal of Water, Sanitation and Hygiene for Development*, *7*(2), 272–289.

Asthana, A. N. (2003). Decentralisation and supply efficiency: The case of rural water supply in central India. *Journal of Development Studies*, *39*(4), 148–159.

Baker, K. K., Story, W. T., Walser-Kuntz, E., & Zimmerman, M. B. (2018). Impact of social capital, harassment of women and girls, and water and sanitation access on premature birth and low infant birth weight in India. *PLoS One*, *13*(10). https://doi.org/10.1371/journal.pone.0205345; https://www.ncbi.nlm.nih.gov/pmc/articles/PMC6175511/

Banda, K., Sarkar, R., Gopal, S., Govindarajan, J., Harijan, B. B., Jeyakumar, M. B., ... Balraj, V. (2007). Water handling, sanitation and defecation practices in rural southern India: A knowledge, attitudes and practices study. *Transactions of the Royal Society of Tropical Medicine and Hygiene*, *101*(11), 1124–1130.

Barnard, S., Routray, P., Majorin, F., Peletz, R., Boisson, S., Sinha, A., & Clasen, T. (2013). Impact of Indian total sanitation campaign on toilet coverage and use: A cross-sectional study in Orissa three years following programme implementation. *PLoS One*, *8*(8), e71438.

Bhallamudi, S. M., Kaviyarasan, R., Abilarasu, A., & Philip, L. (2019). Nexus between sanitation and groundwater quality: Case study from a hard rock region in India. *Journal of Water, Sanitation and Hygiene for Development*, *9*(4), 703–713.

Bicchieri, C. (2016). *Norms in the wild: How to diagnose, measure, and change social norms*. Oxford University Press.

Callahan, D. (1973). The WHO definition of' health. *Hastings Center Studies*, *1*(3), 77–87.

Caruso, B. A., Cooper, H., Haardörfer, R., Yount, K. M., Routray, P., Torondel, B., & Clasen, T. (2018). The association between women's sanitation experiences and mental health: A cross-sectional study in Rural, Odisha India. *SSM - Population Health*, *5*, 257–266. https://doi.org/10.1016/j.ssmph.2018.06.005

Chambers, R., & Von Medeazza, G. (2013). Sanitation and stunting in India: Undernutrition's blind spot. *Economic and Political Weekly*, *48*(25), 15–18.

Chandana, N., & Rao, B. (2021). Status of sustainable sanitation chain in rural, semi-urban, and urban regions: A case study of Maharashtra, India. *Journal of Water, Sanitation and Hygiene for Development*, *11*(1), 112–125.

Coffey, D., & Spears, D. (2017). *Where India goes: Abandoned toilets, stunted development and the costs of caste*. HarperCollins Publishers.

Coffey, D., Gupta, A., Hathi, P., Khurana, N., Spears, D., Srivastav, N., & Vyas, S. (2014). Revealed preference for open defecation. *Economic and Political Weekly*, *49*(38), 43–55.

Coffey, D., Gupta, A., Hathi, P., Spears, D., Srivastav, N., & Vyas, S. (2017a). Understanding open defecation in rural India: Untouchability, pollution, and latrine pits. *Economic and Political Weekly*, *52*(1), 59–66.

Coffey, D., Spears, D., & Vyas, S. (2017b). Switching to sanitation: Understanding latrine adoption in a representative panel of rural Indian households. *Social Science and Medicine*, *188*, 41–50.

Cofie, P., De Allegri, M., Kouyate, B., & Sauerborn, R. (2013). Effects of information, education, and communication campaign on a community-based health insurance scheme in Burkina Faso. *Global Health Action*, *6*(1), 20791.

Crawford, I. M., & Lomas, R. A. (1980). Factory analysis—A tool for data reduction. *European Journal of Marketing*, *14*(7), 414–421.

Cronin, A. A., Prakash, A., Sridhar, P., & Coates, S. (2016). Drinking water supply in India: Context and prospects. In V. Narain & A. Narayanamoorthy (Eds.), *Indian water policy at the crossroads: Resources, technology and reforms, global issues in water policy* (pp. 49–71). Springer. https://doi.org/10.1007/978-3-319-25184-4_4

De, I. (2009). Decentralisation on access to rural water supply services: A study of six villages in West Bengal, India. *Asia-Pacific Journal of Rural Development*, *19*(1), 135–154.

De, I. (2010). Major constraints in the progress of decentralised delivery of rural sanitation programme in West Bengal, India. *IUP Journal of Governance & Public Policy*, *5*(4), 63–83.

De, I. (2018). Determinants of rural sanitation in India and implications for public policy. *Journal of Water, Sanitation and Hygiene for Development*, *8*(4), 650–659.

De, I. (2022). Women's empowerment, work environment, and income: Evidence from India. *Development in Practice*, *32*(4), 468–480.

De, I., & Nag, T. (2016). Dangers of decentralisation in urban slums: A comparative study of water supply and drainage service delivery in Kolkata, India. *Development Policy Review*, *34*(2), 253–276.

De, I., Singh, S., & Panda, S. S. (2021). *Social norms, gender and collective behaviour: Development paradigms in India*. Springer Nature.

Deacon, B., & Olatunji, B. O. (2007). Specificity of disgust sensitivity in the prediction of behavioral avoidance in contamination fear. *Behaviour Research and Therapy*, *45*(9), 2110–2120. https://doi.org/10.1016/j.brat.2007.03.008

Dhaktode, N. (2014). Freedom from open defecation: Role of the community. *Economic and Political Weekly*, 28–30.

Dhanuka, R. K. (2008). *Knowledge, attitude and practice related to sanitation: A household study in the village Unsar PrantI*. IRMA Fieldwork Segment Report (archived). Faculty Guide: Preeti Priya (State: Bihar; District: Muzaffarpur; Village: Pranti).

Dickinson, K. L., Patil, S. R., Pattanayak, S. K., Poulos, C., & Yang, J. H. (2015). Nature's call: Impacts of sanitation choices in Orissa, India. *Economic Development and Cultural Change*, *64*(1), 1–29. https://doi.org/10.3390/ijerph16050734

Dittmer, A. (2009). *Towards total sanitation: Socio-cultural barriers and triggers to total sanitation in West Africa*. WaterAid. https://washmatters.wateraid.org/publications/sanitation/west-africa

Esrey, S. A., Gough, J., Rapapor, D., Sawyer, R., SimpsonHebert, M., Vargas, J., et al. (1998). *Ecological sanitation*. Swedish International Development Cooperation Agency.

Fagbemiro, O. O., Ademuyiwa, I. Y., Soyemi, O. D., & Ojo, A. O. (2016). Factors determining sanitation information-seeking behavior: A literature review. *Tropical Journal of Medical Research*, *19*(2), 81. Retrieved January 2022, from http://www.tjmrjournal.org

Fishbein, M., & Ajzen, A. (1975). *Beliefs, attitudes, intentions, and behavior: An introduction to theory and research*. Addison-Wesley.

George, B. (2009). Sanitation programmes: A glass half-full. *Economic and Political Weekly*, *44*(8), 65–67. http://www.jstor.org/stable/40278531

Gertler, P., Shah, M., Alzua, M. L., Cameron, L., Martinez, S., & Patil, S. (2015). *How does health promotion work? Evidence from the dirty business of eliminating open defecation* (No. w20997). National Bureau of Economic Research.

Ghosh, A., Gupta, A., & Spears, D. (2014). Are children in West Bengal shorter than children in Bangladesh? *Economic and Political Weekly*, 21–24.

GoI. (u.d.). *National urban sanitation: Policy*. Ministry of Urban Development. Government of India. https://www.mohua.gov.in/upload/uploadfiles/files/NUSP_0.pdf

GOI. (2001). *Annual report 2001-02*. Ministry of Rural Development. Retrieved June 22, 2022, from https://rural.nic.in/sites/default/files/AnnualReport2020_21English.pdf

GOM. (1998). Water supply and sanitation department. 1998. "India- Second Maharastra rural water supply sanitation project". *Tribal* (Indigenous People) Development Plan, No. IPP47. http://www-wds.worldbank.org/external/default/WDSContentServer/WDSP/IB/2003/05/30/000094946_03052004071312/Rendered/PDF/multi0page.pdf

Gunyon, W. (1998). *India: Making government funding work harder. A WaterAid report*. Retrieved June 22, 2022, from https://www.ircwash.org/sites/default/files/WaterAid-1998-India.pdf

Gupta, A. S. (2002). National health policy 2002: A brief critique. *National Medical Journal of India*, *15*(4), 215.

Gupta, A. S., Coffey, D., & Spears, D. (2016). *Purity, pollution, and untouchability: Challenges affecting the adoption, use, and sustainability of sanitation programmes in rural India. Sustainable sanitation for all: Experiences, challenges, and innovations* (Vol. 283). Retrieved June 18, 2022, from https://core.ac.uk/download/pdf/286047218.pdf#page=301

Halvorson, S. J., & Wescoat Jr., J. L. (2020). Guarding the sons of empire: Military–state–society relations in water, sanitation and health programs of mid-19th-century India. *Water*, *12*(2), 429. https://doi.org/10.3390/w12020429

Hathi, P., Spears, D., & Coffey, D. (2016). Can collective action strategies motivate behaviour change to reduce open defecation in rural India? *Waterlines*, *35*(2), 118–135. http://www.jstor.org/stable/26600730

Hart-Davis, A. (2008). *Thunder, flush and Thomas Crapper: An encyclopedia*. Michael O'Mara Books.

Harter, M., Contzen, N., & Inauen, J. (2019). The role of social identification for achieving an open-defecation free environment: A cluster-randomized, controlled trial of

Community-Led Total Sanitation in Ghana. *Journal of Environmental Psychology*, *66*, 101360.

Heckman, J. J. (2007). The economics, technology, and neuroscience of human capability formation. *Proceedings of the National Academy of Sciences*, *104*(33), 13250–13255.

Hoddinott, J., Alderman, H., Behrman, J. R., Haddad, L., & Horton, S. (2013). The economic rationale for investing in stunting reduction. *Maternal & Child Nutrition*, *9*, 69–82.

https://jalshakti-ddws.gov.in/sites/default/files/201906_SBM_IEC_Whitepaper.pdf.

https://swachhbharatmission.gov.in/SBMCMS/writereaddata/Portal/Images/pdf/NARSS_2017-18_Report.pd

Iyer, P. (1998, May 5–8). *Uttar Pradesh State, India: The Swajal project, experiences with implementing a demand- responsive approach*. Paper Presented at the Community Water Supply and Sanitation Conference. The World Bank, Washington, DC.

Jain, A., Fernald, L. C., Smith, K. R., & Subramanian, S. V. (2019). Sanitation in rural India: Exploring the associations between dwelling space and household latrine ownership. *International Journal of Environmental Research and Public Health*, *16*(5), 734.

Jenkins, M. W., & Curtis, V. (2005). Achieving the 'good life': Why some people want latrines in rural Benin. *Social Science and Medicine*, *61*(11), 2446–2459. https://doi.org/10.1016/j.socscimed.2005.04.036

Jenkins, M. W., & Scott, B. (2007). Behavioral indicators of household decision-making and demand for sanitation and potential gains from social marketing in Ghana. *Social Science and Medicine*, *64*(12), 2427–2442. https://doi.org/10.1016/j.socscimed.2007.03.010

Jewitt, S. (2011). Geographies of shit Spatial and temporal variations in attitudes towards human waste. *Progress in Human Geography*, *35*(5), 608–626.

Joshi, P. C., & Khattri, P. (2019). On Gandhi and sanitation. *Journal of the Anthropological Survey of India*, *68*(2), 210–224.

Kabeer, N. (1999). Resources, agency, achievements: Reflections on the measurement of women's empowerment. *Development and Change*, *30*(3), 435–464.

Kaliski, J. (2015). *The past, present, and future of sanitation, with a case study of India: Where and why we should give a sh* t* (Doctoral dissertation). Amherst College. Retrieved January 2022, from https://indiawaterweek.thewaternetwork.com/document-XAs/the-past-present-and-future-of-sanitation-with-a-case-study-of-india-3NK00NnqFDfT2pJbD2jo_Q

Kar, K., & Chambers, R. (2008). *Handbook on community-led total sanitation*. Retrieved June 18, 2022, from http://ndr.mw:8080/xmlui/bitstream/handle/123456789/1191/Handbook%20on%20Community-Led%20Total%20Sanitation.pdf?sequence=1

Khan, S., Angelakis, A., & Rose, J. (2014). Sanitation and wastewater technologies in Harappa/Indus valley civilization (ca. 2600–1900 BC). In. A. N. Angelakis & J. B. Rose (Eds.), *Evolution of sanitation and wastewater technologies through the centuries* (pp. 25–42). IWA Publishing.

Khanna, T., & Das, M. (2016). Why gender matters in the solution towards safe sanitation? Reflections from rural India. *Global Public Health*, *11*(10), 1185–1201.

Kumar, A. (2015). Discrepancies in sanitation statistics of rural India. *Economic and Political Weekly*, *50*(2), 13–15.

Leary, V. A. (1994). The right to health in international human rights law. *Health and Human Rights*, *1*(1), 24–56. https://doi.org/10.2307/4065261

Lee, Y. J. (2017). Informing women and improving sanitation: Evidence from rural India. *Journal of Rural Studies*, *55*, 203–215.

Leong, C. (2020). Narratives of sanitation: Motivating toilet use in India. *Geoforum*, *111*, 24–38. https://doi.org/10.1016/j.geoforum.2019.10.001

Lüthi, D. (2010). Private cleanliness, public mess: Purity, pollution and space in Kottar, South India. *Urban Pollution: Cultural Meanings, Social Practices*, *15*, 57–85.

MacFarlane, A. (2003). *The savage war of peace*. Palgrave MacMillan.

Makumbe, J. (1996). *Participatory development: The case of Zimbabwe*. University of Zimbabwe Publications.

Malhotra, N. K., Kim, S. S., & Agarwal, J. (2004). Internet users' information privacy concerns (IUIPC): The construct, the scale, and a causal model. *Information Systems Research*, *15*(4), 336–355.

Mara, D., Lane, J., Scott, B., & Trouba, D. (2010). Sanitation and health. *PLoS Medicine*, *7*(11), e1000363. https://doi.org/10.1371/journal.pmed.1000363

McGranahan, G. (2015). Realizing the right to sanitation in deprived urban communities: Meeting the challenges of collective action, coproduction, affordability, and housing tenure. *World Development*, *68*, 242–253.

McKee, N., Becker-Benton, A., & Bockh, E. (2014). Social and behavior change communication. In K. G. Wilkins, T. Tufte, & R. Obregon (Eds.), *The handbook of development communication and social change* (pp. 278–297). John Wiley & Sons, Inc.

Mehta, M. (2018). Public finance at scale for rural sanitation–a case of Swachh Bharat mission, India. *Journal of Water, Sanitation and Hygiene for Development*, *8*(3), 359–373.

Ministry of Drinking Water and Sanitation. (2019). *Sanitation An assessment of the reach and value of IEC activities under Swachh Bharat mission (Grameen): white paper*. Retrieved June 18, 2022, from https://jalshakti-ddws.gov.in/sites/default/files/201906_SBM_IEC_Whitepaper.pdf

Ministry of Drinking Water and Sanitation. (n.d.). *National annual rural sanitation survey (NARSS) 2017–18*. Retrieved June 18, 2022, from https://jalshakti-ddws.gov.in/sites/default/files/NARSS_2017_18.pdf

Mtisi, S., & Nicol, A. (2003). Water points and water policies: Decentralisation and community management in Sangwe communal area, Zimbabwe, sustainable livelihood in Southern Africa. *Research Paper*, *15*. https://www.ids.ac.uk/projects/sustainable-livelihoods-in-southern-africa/

National Statistical Commission. (n.d.). *Annual report 2016-17*. Retrieved June 18, 2022, from https://mospi.gov.in/documents/213904/0/nsc_AR_2016-17.pdf/b4eb2249-bd7d-fd86-67c7-ada219cb64db?t=1595170355439

Novotný, J., Ficek, F., Hill, J. K., & Kumar, A. (2018). Social determinants of environmental health: A case of sanitation in rural Jharkhand. *Science of the Total Environment*, *643*, 762–774.

O'Reilly, K., & Dhanju, R. (2014). Public taps and private connections: The production of caste distinction and common sense in a Rajasthan drinking water supply project. *Transactions of the Institute of British Geographers*, *39*(3), 373–386.

O'Reilly, K., & Louis, E. (2014). The toilet tripod: Understanding successful sanitation in rural India. *Health & Place*, *29*, 43–51.

O'Rourke, E. (1992). The international drinking water supply and sanitation decade: Dogmatic means to a debatable end. *Water Science and Technology*, *26*(7–8), 1929–1939.

Orgill-Meyer, J., Pattanayak, S. K., Chindarkar, N., Dickinson, K. L., Panda, U., Rai, S., ... Jeuland, M. (2019). Long-term impact of a community-led sanitation campaign in India, 2005–2016. *Bulletin of the World Health Organization*, *97*(8), 523–533A. http://doi.org/10.2471/BLT.18.221572.

Ostrom, E. (1990). *Governing the commons: The evolution of institutions for collective action*. Cambridge University Press.

Othman, Z. (2017). *An analysis of the evolution of the world's toilet habits* [Working Paper].

Panda, R. K., & Padhi, G. (2017). Access and usage of home toilets among rural and urban slum households in Odisha: A study. *Review of Management*, *7*(1–2), 9–21.

Patil, S. R., Arnold, B. F., Salvatore, A. L., Briceno, B., Ganguly, S., Colford, J. M. Jr., & Gertler, P. J. (2014). The effect of India's total sanitation campaign on defecation behaviors and child health in rural Madhya Pradesh: A cluster randomized controlled trial. *PLoS Medicine*. https://doi.org/10.1371/journal.pmed.1001709

Patkar, A. (2016). Equality and non-discrimination in sanitation and hygiene: Ensuring the 'one' in everyone. In P. Bongarz, N. Vernon, & J. Fox (Eds.), *Sustainable sanitation for all: Experiences, challenges, and innovations* (pp. 267–280). Practical Action Publishing.

Pattanayak, S. K., Yang, J. C., Dickinson, K. L., Poulos, C., Patil, S. R., Mallick, R. K., ... Praharaj, P. (2009). Shame or subsidy revisited: Social mobilization for sanitation in Orissa, India. *Bulletin of the World Health Organization*, *87*(8), 580–587.

Pushpangadan, K., & Murugan, G. (1998, April 4). User financing and collective action, relevance for sustainable rural water supply in India. *Economic and Political Weekly*, 793–798.

Planning Commission. (2013). *Evaluation study on total sanitation campaign - Volume II*. Programme Evaluation Organization. Planning Commission, Government of India. http://164.100.161.239/reports/peoreport/peo/rep_tscv2_2205.pdf

Qamar, A. H. (2015). 05'Laj', the concept for honor, shame and modesty of a women in Indian popular culture. *Journal of Gender and Social Issues*, *14*(1), 69–84.

Queensland University of Technology, Brisbane Australia. https://eprints.qut.edu.au /109483/

Ramasubban, R. (2008). History of public health in modern India (1857–2005). In M. J. Lewis & K. K. MacPherson (Eds.), *Public health in Asia and pacific: Historical and comparative perspective*. Routledge.

Ramaswamy, G. (2005). *India stinking: Manual scavengers in Andhra Pradesh and their work*. Navayana.

Rao, S. M., Sekhar, M., & Rao, P. R. (2013). Impact of pit-toilet leachate on groundwater chemistry and role of vadose zone in removal of nitrate and E. coli pollutants in Kolar District, Karnataka, India. *Environmental Earth Sciences*, *68*(4), 927–938.

Ravallion, M. (2008, October 25–31). A global perspective on poverty in India. *Economic and Political Weekly*, *43*(43), 31–37.

Routray, P., Torondel, B., Clasen, T., & Schmidt, W.-P. (2017). Women's role in sanitation decision making in rural coastal Odisha, India. *PLoS One*, *12*(5), e0178042. https://doi .org/10.1371/journal. pone.0178042.

Sanyal, P. (2009). From credit to collective action: The role of microfinance in promoting women's social capital and normative influence. *American Sociological Review*, *74*(4), 529–550.

Sarkar, S. K., & Bharat, G. K. (2021). Achieving sustainable development goals in water and sanitation sectors in India. *Journal of Water, Sanitation and Hygiene for Development*, *11*(5), 693–705.

Schmidt, W. P. (2014). The elusive effect of water and sanitation on the global burden of disease. *Tropical Medicine & International Health*, *19*(5), 522–527.

Schnall, S., Benton, J., & Harvey, S. (2008). With a clean conscience: Cleanliness reduces the severity of moral judgments. *Psychological Science*, *19*(12), 1219–1222.

Scholder, S. V. H. K., Smith, G. D., Lawlor, D. A., Propper, C., & Windmeijer, F. (2013). Child height, health and human capital: Evidence using genetic markers. *European Economic Review*, *57*, 1–22.

Sclar, G. D., Penakalapati, G., Caruso, B. A., Rehfuess, E. A., Garn, J. V., Alexander, K. T., ... Clasen, T. (2018). Exploring the relationship between sanitation and mental and social wellbeing: A systematic review and qualitative synthesis. *Social Science & Medicine, 217*, 121–134.

Seetharam, K. (2015). Challenges and opportunities for sanitation in developing countries. *Journal of Science Policy & Governance, 7*(1). https://www.sciencepolicyjournal.org/uploads/5/4/3/4/5434385/seetharam-jspg-issue7.pdf

Sharma, A., Aasaavari, A., & Anand, S. (2015). Understanding issues involved in toilet access for women. *Economic and Political Weekly, 50*(34), 70–74.

Shweder, R. A., Much, N. C., Mahapatra, M., & Park, L. (1997). The "Big Three" of morality (autonomy, community, and divinity) and the "big three" explanations of suffering. In A. Brandt & P. Rozin (Eds.), *Morality and health* (pp. 119–169). Routledge.

Sifaki, E. (2019). Women's work and agency in GPNS during economic crises: The case of the Greek table grapes export sector. *Feminist Economics, 25*(3), 70–95.

Singh, V., Phuleria, H. C., & Chandel, M. K. (2020). Estimation of energy recovery potential of sewage sludge in India: Waste to watt approach. *Journal of Cleaner Production, 276*, 122538.

Slaymaker, T., & Peter, N. (2004). *Implication of water supply & sanitation programmes under PRSPs, ODI, water policy programme*.

Speltini, G., & Passini, S. (2014). Cleanliness/dirtiness, purity/impurity as social and psychological issues. *Culture and Psychology, 20*(2), 203–219. https://doi.org/10.1177/1354067X14526895

Sorensen, J. P. R., Sadhu, A., Sampath, G., Sugden, S., Gupta, S. D., Lapworth, D. J., ... Pedley, S. (2016). Are sanitation interventions a threat to drinking water supplies in rural India? An application of tryptophan-like fluorescence. *Water Research, 88*, 923–932.

Spears, D. (2020). Exposure to open defecation can account for the Indian enigma of child height. *Journal of Development Economics, 146*, 102277. https://doi.org/10.1016/j.jdeveco.2018.08.003

Spears, D., Ghosh, A., & Cumming, O. (2013). Correction: Open defecation and childhood stunting in India: An ecological analysis of new data from 112 districts. *PLoS One, 8*(9), e73784. https://doi.org/10.1371/annotation/9ffcb740-f394-41af-bbbc-800c7cc25ea8

Srinivas, T. (2002). Flush with success: Bathing, defecation, worship, and social change in South India. *Space and Culture, 5*(4), 368–386. https://doi.org/10.1177/1206331202005004004

Thaler, R. H., & Sunstein, C. R. (2008). *Nudge: Improving decisions about health, wealth, and happiness*. Yale University Press.

Tiwary, S. K., & Saurabh, S. (2018). Archaeological evidences of toilet system in ancient India. *Heritage: Journal of Multidisciplinary Studies in Archaeology, 6*, 764–781.

van der Geest, S. (1998). Akan shit: Getting rid of dirt in Ghana. *Anthropology Today, 14*(3), 8–12.

Van Vliet, B. J. M., Spaargaren, G., & Oosterveer, P. (2010). Introduction. In B. J. M. Van Vliet, G. Spaargaren, & P. Oosterveer (Eds.), *Social Perspectives on the Sanitation Challenge* (pp. 1–8). Springer.

Veerashekharappa. (2000, February 12–18). Reforms in rural drinking water supply. *Economic and Political Weekly, 35*(7). https://www.epw.in/journal/2000/07/discussion/reforms-rural-drinking-water-supply.html.

Vyas, S., & Spears, D. (2018). Sanitation and religion in South Asia: What accounts for differences across countries? *The Journal of Development Studies, 54*(11), 2119–2135.

Wasonga, J., Okowa, M., & Kioli, F. (2016). Sociocultural determinants to adoption of safe water, sanitation, and hygiene practices in Nyakach, Kisumu County, Kenya: A descriptive qualitative study. *Journal of Anthropology, 2016.* http://dx.doi.org/10.1155/2016/7434328

Waterkeyn, J., & Cairncross, S. (2005). Creating demand for sanitation and hygiene through Community Health Clubs: A cost-effective intervention in two districts in Zimbabwe. *Social Science and Medicine, 61*(9), 1958–1970. https://doi.org/10.1016/j.socscimed.2005.04.012

Weis, D., Hutton, G., & Kumar, M. (2019). Health costs and benefits from a pilot rural sanitation intervention in India. *Journal of Water, Sanitation and Hygiene for Development, 9*(1), 129–138.

World Health Organization. (2009a). *Diarrhoea: Why children are still dying and what can be done.* https://apps.who.int/iris/bitstream/handle/10665/44174/9789241598415_eng.pdf

World Health Organization. (2009b). *World health statistics 2009.* https://www.who.int/publications/i/item/9789241563819

World Health Organization. (2017). *Diarrhoeal disease.* Retrieved June 23, 2023, from https://www.who.int/news-room/fact-sheets/detail/diarrhoeal-disease

World Bank. (n.d.). *GDP per capita, PPP (current international $).* Retrieved November 23, 2023, from https://data.worldbank.org/indicator/NY.GDP.PCAP.PP.CD

World Bank. (n.d.). *GDP per capita, PPP (current international $).* Retrieved June 23, 2023, from https://data.worldbank.org/indicator/NY.GDP.PCAP.PP.CD

World Bank. (1998a). *Rural water supply and sanitation report, India- water resources management sector review.* World Bank.

World Bank. (1998b). India impact evaluation report, comparative review of rural water systems experience. *Operation Evaluation Department*, Report No. 18114. Retrieved June 22, 2022, from https://documents1.worldbank.org/curated/en/674481468772491925/pdf/multi0page.pdf; Retrieved June 23, 2022, from https://documents1.worldbank.org/curated/ru/961101468050655724/pdf/416730PUB0NO0P1x327349B01PUBLIC1pdf.pdf

WSP. (2003, September). *Governance and financing of water supply and sanitation in Ethiopia, Kenya and South Africa: A cross country synthesis* (Sector Finance Working Papers: No. 5). WSP.

WSP-Water and Sanitation Programme. (2004, May 25–27). Rural water supply and sanitation in Africa global learning process on scaling up poverty reduction, shanghai conference. WSP-Water and Sanitation Programme. Retrieved June 23, 2023, from https://www.ircwash.org/sites/default/files/WSP-2004-Rural.pdf

Zuin, V., Delaire, C., Peletz, R., Cock-Esteb, A., Khush, R., & Albert, J. (2019). Policy diffusion in the rural sanitation sector: Lessons from community-led total sanitation (CLTS). *World Development, 124*, 104643.

Annexure

Regression Models

The dependent variables regarding access to toilets are the following:

$no\_access = 1$, if no access to toilet

0, otherwise

$exclusive\_toilet = 1$, if toilet for exclusive use available

0, otherwise

The dependent variables pertaining to use of toilets are the following:

$use\_male\_below15 = 1$, if toilet used by male below 15 years

0, otherwise

$use\_male\_above15 = 1$, if toilet used by male above 15 years

0, otherwise

$use\_female\_below15 = 1$, if toilet used by female below 15 years

0, otherwise

$use\_female\_above15 = 1$, if toilet used by female above 15 years

0, otherwise

$use\_old = 1$, if toilet used by old members

0, otherwise

$use\_all = 1$, if toilet used by all members of household

0, otherwise

The independent variables explaining all the above-mentioned dependent variables are same as follows:

tot_member = total number of the members at the household;
per_female = percentage of female at the household;
female_hh_head = female-headed household;
hh_head_30 = age of the household head less than 30 years;
edu_male: highest education of male members till standard 10th, 10th and above;
edu_female: highest education of female members till standard 10th, 10th and above;
prim_occu_agri = agricultural households (primary occupation agriculture);
prim_occu_nonagri = non-agricultural households (primary occupation non-agriculture);
prim_occu_salary = salaried household (primary occupation service against salary);
religion: Hindu household as the control variable
drink_water = access to the primary source of drinking water for household's exclusive use;
insuffi_water = insufficient water for all the households' chores throughout the year;
dist_drink_water = the distance travelled to fetch drinking water as inside dwelling, outside dwelling but within the premise, outside premises: less than 400 metres, 400 metres and above;
facility_bathroom = detached or no bathroom;
floor_kuccha = the structure of floor made of mud;
wall_pucca = the structure of the wall made of pucca material;
pucca material includes burnt brick/stone/limestone, iron or other metal sheet, or cement/RBC/RCC;
total_land = land possessed by the household
total_expenses = total expenses of the households;
expense_durgood = percentage of expenses on durable goods and entertainment;
no_aware_SBM = no awareness of SBM at the household;
no_influ_self = construction of toilet not influenced by self;
no_influ_spouse = the construction of the toilet is not influenced by spouse;
years_toilet = number of years passed since construction of toilet till the year 2018;
toilet_exclu = access to toilet for exclusive use of household;
govt_subsidy = government subsidy received by the household for the construction of toilet;
no_flies = no problem of flies at the household;
no_stomach_problem = no cases of stomach problem at the household;
no_malaria = no cases of malaria at the household;
no_skin_disease = no cases of skin disease at the household;
no_fever = no cases of fever at the household;
State: Gujarat, Telangana, and Bihar are control variables here.

Models on Access to Toilets

$$
\begin{aligned}
&\text{no\_access} = \\
&\alpha_0 + \alpha_1\ per\_female + \alpha_2\ hh\_head\_30 + \alpha_3\ female\_hh\_head + \alpha_4\ edu\_male \\
&+\alpha_5\ edu\_female + \alpha_6\ prim\_occu\_agri + \alpha_7\ prim\_occu\_nonagri \\
&+\alpha_8\ prim\_occu\_salary + \alpha_9\ religion + \alpha_{10}\ social\_group + \alpha_{11}\ drink\_water \\
&+\alpha_{12}\ insuffi\_water + \alpha_{13}\ dist\_drink\_water + \alpha_{14}\ facility\_bathroom \\
&+\alpha_{15}\ floor\_kuccha + \alpha_{16}\ wall\_pucca + \alpha_{17}\ total\_land + \alpha_{18}\ total\_\exp enses \\
&+\alpha_{19}\ expense\_durgood + \alpha_{20}\ no\_aware\_SBM + \alpha_{21}\ no\_flies \\
&+\alpha_{22}\ no\_stomach\_prob + \alpha_{23}\ no\_malaria + \alpha_{24}\ no\_skin\_dis + \alpha_{25}\ no\_fever \\
&+\alpha_{26}\ state
\end{aligned}
$$

$$
\begin{aligned}
&\text{exclusive\_toilet} = \\
&\alpha_0 + \alpha_1\ per\_female + \alpha_2\ hh\_head\_30 + \alpha_3\ female\_hh\_head + \alpha_4\ edu\_male \\
&+\alpha_5\ edu\_female + \alpha_6\ prim\_occu\_agri + \alpha_7\ prim\_occu\_nonagri \\
&+\alpha_8\ prim\_occu\_salary + \alpha_9\ religion + \alpha_{10}\ social\_group + \alpha_{11}\ drink\_water \\
&+\alpha_{12}\ insuffi\_water + \alpha_{13}\ dist\_drink\_water + \alpha_{14}\ facility\_bathroom \\
&+\alpha_{15}\ floor\_kuccha + \alpha_{16}\ wall\_pucca + \alpha_{17}\ total\_land + \alpha_{18}\ total\_expenses \\
&+\alpha_{19}\ expense\_durgood + \alpha_{20}\ no\_aware\_SBM + \alpha_{21}\ no\_flies \\
&+\alpha_{22}\ no\_stomach\_prob + \alpha_{23}\ no\_malaria + \alpha_{24}\ no\_skin\_dis + \alpha_{25}\ no\_fever \\
&+\alpha_{26}\ state
\end{aligned}
$$

Models on Use of Toilets

toilet_use =

$$\alpha_0 + \alpha_1\, per\_female + \alpha_2\, hh\_head\_30 + \alpha_3\, female\_hh\_head + \alpha_4\, edu\_male$$
$$+\alpha_5\, edu\_female + \alpha_6\, prim\_occu\_agri + \alpha_7\, prim\_occu\_nonagri$$
$$+\alpha_8\, prim\_occu\_salary + \alpha_9\, religion + \alpha_{10}\, tot\_member + \alpha_{11}\, drink\_water$$
$$+\alpha_{12}\, insuffi\_water + \alpha_{13}\, dist\_drink\_water + \alpha_{14}\, facility\_bathroom$$
$$+\alpha_{15}\, floor\_kuccha + \alpha_{16}\, wall\_pucca + \alpha_{17}\, total\_land + \alpha_{18}\, total\_expenses$$
$$+\alpha_{19}\, expense\_durgood + \alpha_{20}\, no\_aware\_SBM + \alpha_{21}\, no\_\inf lu - self$$
$$+\alpha_{22}\, no\_influ\_spouse + \alpha_{23}\, yrs\_toilet + \alpha_{24}\, toilet\_exclu + \alpha_{25}\, govt\_subsidy$$
$$+\alpha_{26}\, no\_stomach\_prob + \alpha_{27}\, no\_malaria + \alpha_{28}\, no\_skin\_dis + \alpha_{29}\, no\_flies$$
$$+\alpha_{30}\, no\_fever + \alpha_{31}\, state$$

	use_male_below15	**(use of toilet among male below 15 years)**
	use_male_above15	(use of toilet among male above 15 years)
where toilet_use =	**use_female_below15**	**(use of toilet among female below 15 years)**
	use_female_above15	(use of toilet among female above 15 years)
	use_old	(use of toilet by old)
	use_all	(use of toilet by all)

Index

www.ingramcontent.com/pod-product-compliance
Ingram Content Group UK Ltd.
Pitfield, Milton Keynes, MK11 3LW, UK
UKHW022020180926
475701UK00005B/948
* 9 7 8 1 0 3 2 7 2 6 2 5 0 *